Cancer Was
My Companion

Cancer Was My Companion

A Memoir

David I Brown

Sorrell Books

Published 2017 by SORRELL BOOKS

6 3 2 5 7 4 6 5 0 8

ISBN: 978-1548074326

Introduction

I reached the comfort of late middle age with little or no experience of illness in all of my adult life. I had a loving wife, Grace, a beautiful new home which nestled at the foot of the Chiltern Hills in Buckinghamshire and a bolt-hole right next to the sea in West Sussex. Weekends away were exhilarating and uplifting; we loved the sea and the coastline. I was proud of my three daughters who were furthering their academic studies, developing their careers and becoming independent.

I had a new career, having started up my own consultancy business not long before. Although the work was challenging and tough, it was also hugely enjoyable and fulfilling.

Then I was told I had cancer.

It hit me like a freight train; I knew I could die. I underwent treatment, including major surgery. Then, only a few months later, when I thought I'd got it beaten, I found out I had secondary cancer. This time, dying seemed inevitable.

It was the worst time of my life. The physical pain and the medical procedures that I needed to endure to overcome my condition drove me almost to despair.

But I got through it. Somehow, I survived with the help of many people – family, friends and medics. Now I'm rebuilding my life. I know how unlucky I was and how lucky I am. Looking back on it all it's hard to believe what happened, how many people it affected and just how much of my life I lost in the process.

Afterwards, I just knew I needed to tell my story, not just the technicalities of the illness and its treatment but, more importantly, the emotionally savage path it took me down.

If, when I was first diagnosed with cancer, I had known someone who had been through it all as I have, perhaps their story would have helped me cope that little bit better. Perhaps my story could perform that role for other people. I began to write with the aim of helping others who confront challenges like mine.

One thing I know, however much I hated it and however much I fought and conquered it, cancer will always be my companion, the demon on my shoulder.

There are some people I would like to thank: My adorable wife Grace who has been my rock; my three wonderful girls for their constant support and love; my close friends who were always there for me and especially the radiotherapy and chemotherapy nurses, my consultant oncologist and the amazing liver surgeons who messed with my insides. Without all these people's help I wouldn't be alive today to write this.

Special thanks to my editor William Peskett for his patience and wisdom, freely given, and to the artist Marion Coutts whose memoir *Iceberg* gave me emotional inspiration.

Chapter 1

Returning home from my latest arduous business trip to India, I was feeling tired and, well, generally under the weather. I was already overdue for my regular check-up by the company doctor and so, seeing an opportunity to get a thorough examination, I made an appointment.

It was early July 2010. The company doctor performed all the usual tests: he measured my blood pressure and my resting heartbeat; he peered into my nose, throat and ears; and of course he took a blood sample. As the blood was drawn out, it crossed my mind with discomfort that the doctor would shortly discover my cholesterol level. I knew it would be higher than the recommended figure, but then isn't everyone's?

Blood pressure systolic 140 over diastolic 78: high but still in the normal range. I was told I should think twice before eating fatty foods. Heartbeat at rest 65: normal.

I left the clinic feeling as positive as a 57-year-old man can after such an ordeal.

Two days later I was called back. The company doctor looked more serious than before. It was bad news about my cholesterol. My levels were too high. I measured 7.0mmol/l for total cholesterol, with HDL (good cholesterol) at 1.5mmol/l – a good result – but LDL (bad cholesterol) at a worrying 5.5mmol/l. A healthy adult should have an LDL level under 3.0mmol/l. I was told to get my LDL bad cholesterol level down under 5.0 straight away. I should see my GP; I should probably take some statins. Perhaps I should be screened for stress. Every business trip to India caused me stress. Trips like that would cause anyone stress. It was the travel, the traffic, the poverty, the rich, exotic food and of course the beer.

My family was all there and as always we felt together as one, even though those days the girls, Emily the eldest and the twins Harriet and Alice, were really actually elsewhere – their school education completed and degrees done, jobs found; they had all moved out but came home often. Grace, my wife, was there as always. She is my constant.

Our home is our Colosseum, where battles may take place – some won and some lost – but most are agreed amicably. Festivals and festivities, laughter and love are all part of our lives here. Our home is where we can be ourselves, where we are relaxed and content away from the world and its troubles, happy in our own lives and our own world.

It would all change soon, this happy dynamic, especially my part in it. Something was to come to destroy our happiness, cracking open its solidity and strength, bringing in those troubles that we thought existed only in the outside world.

I went to see my GP who looked at my cholesterol levels with a professional air and prescribed statins, to be taken daily and to start immediately. Did I need to change my diet? No, there was no need as the magic pills would do the job.

I have two issues about food. First, I like it, and second, I can eat more than is good for me. Also I have an issue about alcohol: I drink too much. It's not that I am fat or even overweight. I measure five foot 10 inches (1.78m) and weigh a reasonable 12 stone (76.2kg). However, when it comes to unhealthy eating, my diet is extreme compared with Grace's for example. I often have a full English breakfast which Grace would never do. It's usually yogurt and fruit for her and cereal and bacon for me. At dinner, give me gravy and a sauce, puddings the English way. Ice cream or custard. Fricassee.

In our house, Grace is in charge of weight loss. It is her area of authority and knowledge, determination and capability. Mine is addiction. I have an addictive nature. I smoked from the age of 15, only giving it up when I was in my mid-50s. It was the vicar's son who taught me how to smoke. He was my friend and we'd smoke in his tree house. In those days the cigarette brands were *Guards* and *Player's No 6*. Then a French friend started me on *Gitanes*. I liked whisky too; oh, and wine.

Grace will have no salt, no saturated fat and no cream. She eats little butter, choosing margarine instead. She takes smaller portions and leaves out the chips. Perhaps I would be OK if I ate off smaller plates. I should put a sign on the front of the fridge, "Not today you won't".

No is an absolute. It means what it says.

Except that I have an addictive nature.

After a few weeks I made a follow-up visit to my GP. My cholesterol level had fallen but I would need to go on taking the pills, maybe forever, to ensure that my bad cholesterol level behaved itself and stayed low. I felt generally better about my health except that my bowel movements had changed and I reported my concern. I was a little "looser" as the doctor repeated back to me, the way doctors do. It's expected, he said. It's what happens, he said. It will settle down, get back to normal, he said finally.

A few months later, things hadn't got back to normal. I left it for six months before I went to see my GP again. He suggested a different type of statin, from a different pharmaceutical manufacturer. From a chemical point of view I never did see the logic in this, but like most people I thought doctors were supposed to know what they were talking about. What did I know? OK, my degree was science based but I was no medic.

Another six months passed and my situation wasn't improving. In fact it was getting worse and still I thought the cause lay elsewhere. It was at this time that my company reorganised, as companies do, my role was declared redundant and I found myself out of a job. However, I managed to find another position within weeks and felt happy that I had beaten all those 30-something applicants to the job. This was to be my new start, a new role as a consultant with a well-regarded analytical laboratory. Even though I was very pleased to get the job, from the first day when I walked through those old aluminium-and-glass swing doors into that tired blue-and-grey reception area, with its polystyrene-tiled ceiling and fake leather-clad reception desk, I knew I was going to hate every single day.

And I did.

Was I suffering from stress again or was it something worse? If I was stressed, then my brain wasn't providing me with all the right information. Or was it lying to me? Maybe my body was telling me the truth but my brain was hiding the information.

Either way, the truth was about to come out.

Chapter 2

Team GB did brilliantly at the 2012 London Olympics, winning 65 medals. London is the only city to host the Games three times and the country was buzzing with excitement. Grace and I had been up to take in the atmosphere in the Olympic village before it all started. We also watched the Olympic torch scurry through Waddesdon where the route came nearest to our village. There were a lot of people waving flags and drinking beer, a lot of traffic and coaches. The torch came and then, whoosh, it was gone.

I got the T-shirt though and wore it proudly.

We were looking forward to the Paralympics that were to follow the main Games. Our daughter Harriet was involved in these as she was working in marketing for the local council. The Paralympics were first held in 1948, for injured war veterans. The inaugural event took place in the grounds of Stoke Mandeville Hospital in Aylesbury, only seven miles from our village. The track is still there today, close to the hospital's world-renowned spinal unit. A very dear friend of ours worked at Stoke Mandeville and spent a lot of time there after a supposedly simple operation, done at another hospital at age 14, went wrong and left her paralysed from the waist down and in a wheel chair for the rest of her life. Emily, our eldest daughter, worked there too, spending time in both the burns and cancer units before she fully qualified as a clinical psychologist and again after gaining her doctorate from Oxford University in 2014. But that was later, not now, not when the Olympics were in London for the third time, not before the Paralympics were about to start.

For me it began during the night with some abdominal pain and a fever that lasted the weekend. Grace called our local medical centre and spoke to a doctor, who immediately prescribed the usual medication and said that if I hadn't improved by Monday, we were to call him again.

I didn't improve. When Grace called him back he told us he was concerned. It was probably diverticulitis but he wanted a second opinion. I should report to the accident and emergency department at our nearest hospital. Within an hour we were sitting among many others in a very full A&E department. Hours slipped by and I began to feel more unwell. If you have eight hours to kill, a National Health Service (NHS) A&E department is not the best place to be at the best of times. I looked around my fellow patients: old people with weekend ailments; young people too drunk to remember how not to fall off a child's trampoline. A teenager was squealing and swearing that his ankle was broken. He hobbled in to see the triage nurse whimpering and came out laughing that his ankle was only sprained.

Then I was summoned to see the triage nurse myself. I don't remember much of what happened. Questions, I remember being asked many questions. What was my name, age, occupation and address, my name and age, my name? I was to be asked these same questions many times by many different members of the medical staff. Nurses, staff nurses, auxiliary nurses, doctors, registrars, consultants, more nurses and yet more nurses, again and again in many different places, wards, beds, clinics, surgeries, ante-rooms, preparation rooms, assessment centres, waiting rooms, receptions, more hospital beds, on trolleys, off trolleys, on chairs, on sofas. Every time the information was written down in little books, black books, big red books, on proformas, on pink or green forms, on note pads and many times tapped into computers.

I could tell it wasn't good. I was prodded by a young doctor, new to the game. He was nice and kind but perhaps a little naïve.

Suddenly it was time for a computerised tomography (CT) scan. Things escalated quickly. The situation became traumatic and before I knew it I was being taken into surgery. I was to have something removed from my body by laparoscopic (keyhole) surgery.

When I came round I was screaming in agony. I remember swearing a lot. The f-word was freely vomited from my mouth as my arms were held down by two young nurses with bright eyes and determined looks. I think a morphine-rich needle was stuck in me somewhere as suddenly the pain began to subside – alarmingly quickly in fact. I stopped swearing and the nurses let go of my arms. I lay there shivering in my backless, bloodied and fouled gown for a while until I felt myself suddenly being moved into another room. This was a blue, lit space where I was stripped, re-clothed and trolleyed somewhere else before I finally closed my eyes to sleep.

The operation had been a success, I was told. I could go home but not yet, I was told, not until I had eaten my egg sandwich and drunk my orange juice, neither of which I wanted. A thirty-something-year-old nurse in a blue uniform with folded arms and an attitude about obeying rules – her rules – stood over me. I decided she had always wanted to be a doctor but didn't have the brains for it. She certainly had the attitude and the balls but perhaps not the brains or the finesse. Just because the doctor said I could go home didn't mean that I could get dressed, phone my wife or pack my bag. What I had to do was eat my egg sandwich, drink my orange juice and allow Nurse Attitude to dictate the terms of my release to me.

Eventually I was allowed to go home. Despite the pain, I was relieved that whatever it was that was causing my condition had been sorted out. I had a couple of small holes in me, one where a drain tube had been inserted and had fallen out and another through which the laparoscopic surgery had been performed. These scarred my abdomen and, although they were a little sore, I felt that I would easily manage. The problem was that by the following weekend the fever had returned and I spent another night in soaking sheets and racked with a painful fire in my head. Grace called out the local doctor as an emergency. He actually came!

I was back in A&E.

This time I was sent straight past the queues of patients to the A&E ward, which was strange. It was just the other side of a very busy unit. I stayed in that dark, strange environment for two nights. No beds, just trolleys. It was like a road junction with traffic lights at which we on our trolleys were all waiting for the off. When a bed on a ward became available, the green light flashed on and one of us would be zoomed off to claim it. For two days I watched others getting their green light. We missed Nick's daughter's wedding, so he came with Grace to see me there, parked at the dingy traffic junction on my trolley, waiting my turn for a green light.

It was quite weird.

Another emergency was about to take place. There were more CT scans and magnetic resonance imaging (MRI) scans and prodding and x-raying. This time, the decision was to perform another laparoscopy, but inside the CT scanner, under a local anaesthetic and sedatives. The point of this operation was to sew up the hole that had been made during my first operation. The drainage probe had been put into my small intestine instead of my abdomen. Well a mistake like that can be made by any top surgical team. Not that I knew any of this at the time or even just after; not until Grace and I were given conflicting information as to the reason for this follow-up procedure did we start to question what had been done to me. Not until much later when I read my notes together with another doctor did I realise the "mistake" that had been made, the malpractice that no one was to admit to, take the blame for or tell the patient about.

It wasn't until later that I was to uncover the cover-up.

Like all professionals, doctors close ranks when their incompetence results in mistakes. My brother, a dental surgeon, told me the same is true in his world.

Chapter 3

Staying in a ward with five other men shouldn't ordinarily be too much of a problem. Apart from the food, which I won't go into, and the nurses, many of whom were usually either too busy elsewhere or too busy chatting, things were OK on the ward. One Polish male auxiliary nurse who was on duty at night was by far the most caring and competent of the lot.

I wouldn't use those words to describe one of the more senior sisters who, under major duress as it was seemingly below her status, was tasked with taking a blood sample from me. She told me to sit on the chair beside my bed so she could jab away in the general area of my elbow until she found an already-bruised but still viable vein. It hurt like hell, which made me question her level of competence, but what was most disturbing was the amount of blood that was now rapidly escaping from both vein and needle, running copiously down my arm, the arm of the chair and the front chair leg to form a thickening slick of deep red liquid on the floor. Sample taken, I was asked to press on a wad of cotton wool to stem the bleeding as she swaggered off, job done.

That encrusted pool of blood stayed there for a full three days. Each day a tall, dark, male cleaner, whom I imagined to be the head of the cleaners' mafia, somehow missed it when he mopped around all the beds. I decided to see how many days would pass before it was cleaned up but eventually I couldn't bear to see the now brown, blood-stained floor any longer and pointed it out to a doctor. He, who was on his usual rounds with the sisters, nurses and entourage of pale, tired student doctors, could only stare at me tight-lipped as the red mist glowed in his eyes. I was never sure whether he wished that I had died on the operating table or that the sister he had reprimanded should be the next to go under his knife.

Grace came to visit me every day of course. The girls also came when they could. They brought me papers and books and news and get-well wishes. All my family sent me greetings and my sisters came to visit. Some friends came with goodie bags which was great.

During this second recuperation period things started to go wrong inside me again. I was being starved and therefore allowed to take only sips of liquid. They needed my colon to be empty as they took more scans and x-rays. I was losing weight, over two stone (12.7kg) in the end.

I wasn't sleeping well at night. I started having vivid nightmares about milk! For some reason I was desperate for the stuff. I craved it. I would wake in the middle of the night, imagining that I had a glass of milk at the end of the bed but I couldn't reach it. I begged the nurses and even one of the consultants on his rounds the following morning for just one glass of milk. His entourage of students and junior doctors looked at me with horror as if I had asked the consultant for thirty pieces of silver. They brought me no milk. Instead, that night, my wonderful Polish auxiliary nurse brought me a glass of cold water, apologised as that was the best he could do and advised me to close my eyes and just pretend it was milk. I did and it wasn't.

Blood sampling, scanning and prodding went on endlessly but, strangely enough, my mind was kept away from these concerns due to Derek.

Derek was in the bed opposite mine, except that he wasn't actually in a "bed". He kept falling out of his real bed and so had been put on a mattress pushed sideways against the wall. Derek didn't like sheets or blankets, or pyjamas come to think of it. He didn't like doctors and he certainly didn't like sisters. The only member of staff whom Derek seemed to get on with was a Filipino nurse, who used to tuck him in as best she could, lie down with him, give him a cuddle most nights and generally see that he was looked after. This activity probably took up most of her shift. In fact Derek was so needy he probably took up a lot of everyone's shifts.

Derek would constantly shout out that he needed help. "Help me, help me. Oh. come on. Where are you? Come ooonnnnnn," he would wail over and over again until either a nurse actually came or one of us – usually me – pressed the buzzer to summon assistance before we all went crazy and could get some peace and perhaps sleep; at least for half an hour or so until Derek started up again.

Derek's shouting used to provoke a certain female patient in a ward across the corridor who would shout abusive replies that somehow always mirrored Derek's plaintive and woeful wailings.

The most disturbing times were when Derek wanted to go to the toilet, but nobody seemed to understand this nor apparently care. This neglect meant that Derek would throw back his covers, pull down his pyjama bottoms and either defecate or urinate where he lay, all the while screaming for someone to help him.

Derek shouldn't really have been on my ward, the men's ward, Ward 6 at the hospital. Derek had dementia, I was told eventually, having asked many times what his condition was. He had undergone major surgery, but he couldn't go back to his care home as they didn't have the skilled nurses there to look after his post-operative needs. There was nowhere else for him to go so Derek stayed with us on Ward 6 and just lay on his mattress, upset and distressed, confused and lonely except for one little Filipino nurse who was the only person who seemed to care and who used her time and skills to keep him clean, safe and comforted.

At the end of a week of Derek, no food and endless tests, I awoke one morning with a pain in my stomach. It was distended, as if it would burst like a balloon if pricked. I was suddenly scared, despite receiving calming words from several nurses. The doctor was summoned. This time several doctors came in rapid succession and drew the curtains around my bed, reading notes and whispering quietly to each other.

Something had to be done. I had to undergo another operation as the latest CT scan had revealed a blockage in the same place that the first operation had been performed. This was now urgent. They were going to have to remove part of my colon at the junction with my rectum as there seemed to be a blockage and an area that was highly inflamed.

There was no tumour there, they assured me. It was not cancerous. Grace was informed. Preparations were made. Forms were signed. This would be open surgery on the colon. The doctor drew me a picture to make it easier for me to understand what they were going to do. A stoma may be needed and another picture was drawn, again to make it easier for me to comprehend. The stoma may or may not be permanent. Did I understand the consequences? Please sign this consent document agreeing that I understood.

There was also a chance I could die on the operating table. Did I understand that? Please sign this consent document to show that I agreed that I understood.

The trouble was: I understood all too well.

Chapter 4

I awoke to find two lovely and instantly recognisable faces looking down at me. A worried brow or two perhaps, but also smiles, faces showing relief. It was Grace and Emily, our eldest daughter.

The surgeons had removed a third of my colon and fitted a stoma, as a plumber would install a new pipe, attaching it to my gut. Drainage tubes protruded from my abdomen and hung down, a catheter and of course the new addition, a bag like a small balloon stuck on to me at a right angle. This was pink; it was meant to be a skin tone, to make it "blend in". But it was pink as in "pink"! Who has skin that colour? It didn't blend in at all. It bloody well stuck out like a... well, like a bloody bright pink, half-inflated balloon. And it was stuck to me with yet another drainage tube attached.

Looking on the bright side, I hadn't died on the operating table, unless the angels looked exactly like my wife and eldest daughter. Well that would have been okay. I could have "lived" with that.

So I had had a colostomy and the blockage had been removed and I was alive and so we were all relieved.

The doctors visited and the nurses nursed and the surgeon and other consultants came every morning on their rounds, always followed by an entourage of student doctors, all vying for position to listen and learn from the great and wise. They looked worried that they might miss an important part of the diagnosis, prognosis or medical babble that flowed so easily from the consultants' knowledgeable mouths. They pressed closer and scribbled on their pads, eyeing each other's notes to copy anything that they might have missed. I watched the show, the body language of each player. The actors knew their lines well and had good stage presence, although occasionally a student seemed to forget where to stand or when to raise his wavering arm. Not to upstage the top-billing actor, the consultant, was the main aim. Even the sycophantic sisters knew where to stand and how to behave.

I was the object of all their interest. They looked down and checked and prodded and looked again and whispered and the students scribbled and the sisters gazed and talked between themselves and occasionally to a student or the surgeon, but nobody wanted to talk to me, not really talk to me. Yes, they asked if I felt any pain and whether I was feeling woozy, but no one actually asked me how I felt, inside, in my head, in myself. Before I had time to think of the questions I really wanted to ask, they were gone.

What I didn't know at the time, since nobody had told me, was that the thing that had been causing the blockage in my gut was being investigated. Tissue from it had been sent to the pathology laboratory for analysis. They would let me know the results in due course but they were sure that it wasn't a tumour and anyway certainly not malignant. I was to spend another few days recuperating before they could send me home, they said.

Grace came to see me as always and it was so wonderful. The girls came and friends came. I felt that I was at last going to start to get back to some sort of normality, despite the stoma.

Sleeping, especially at night, was proving difficult. The bag attached to my stoma had to be emptied along with all the other vessels that were accumulating my bodily fluids. The "opium" patch stuck on my lower back was obviously running out as the post-operation pain was increasing and general discomfort was preventing me from sleeping deeply for any length of time. I asked for more drugs, any drugs, but I was refused. It seemed that they wanted me to feel the pain!

No pain, no gain. Ha ha!

The following night, I was especially restless. As I lay awake, listening to Derek calling out as usual, an elderly gentleman suddenly arrived on the ward and was wheeled on a bed into the space opposite me. The curtains were drawn but I could hear his wife and two middle-aged children help him get organised, supported by a pair of starchy nurses. After a while they left him to settle for the night.

It wasn't long before I noticed the old man was having difficulty breathing. His wheezes were followed by a coughing fit that left him gasping for air. He hadn't pressed his buzzer; at least no nurse came to attend to him. His breathing became more laboured. I pressed my buzzer and when no one came I pressed it again and again until finally the sister arrived. Her scowl only

25

disappeared when I explained what I could hear taking place in the bed opposite me. What happened next and during the rest of that night will remain with me forever.

The gentleman's breathing became a hoarse rattle. Liquid was building up in his throat and lungs, the sister exclaimed to a new young doctor who had been summoned to the old man's bedside. Although I could hear most of what was going on, it was obvious that they were trying to keep their discussions to a low level, assuming that most other patients on the ward were sleeping. I could hear only the occasional snatches of conversation between the nursing staff and the young duty doctor. The sister suggested that the emergency resuscitation unit should be called at once. This seemed to be ignored as the pack of medical experts left the ward, just like that. The gentleman's breathing sounded worse and became shallower as two nurses returned and again complained in loud whispers that resuscitation experts should be called.

I must have drifted off at this point as suddenly I was fully awake and witness to a flurry of hurried, squeaky footsteps, swishing curtains and raised voices. Through a chink in my curtain I could see a nurse sitting on the old gentleman's body, pumping his chest, calling for support and oxygen, monitors and for the consultant to be called.

The old gentleman died that night. The emergency resuscitation team was never called, despite the persistent demands of the sister on duty. The consultant, when he arrived, called for the man's notes and a moment to read them. There was total silence while he did this. He asked who had made the decisions and was informed by the sister that the young duty doctor had. He closed the note book, asked for the mortuary staff to be called and left along with the duty doctor and nurses. His departing words were, "I'll deal with this; someone call his family."

I lay in my bed and cried, cried for the old gentleman who had been alive just a few hours earlier. I cried for his family who had left him alive just a few hours before that. Cried for his wife who would never again hold his hand and kiss his cheek and whisper, "goodnight, see you in the morning". And I cried for myself and the fact that I had had to listen to what happened and could do nothing. I cried in anger too at the doctor whose inexperience let it happen, at her pride that didn't allow her to open her ears and listen to the sister, and at the consultant whose arrogance and power allowed him to make that decision.

It was almost dawn when the family I had seen just the night before came back. The curtains that had remained closed were quickly parted to allow them to pass into that shrouded place of shame and loss. Tears were shed, quiet, dignified whispers heard and cries muffled in sorrowful respect. The curtains parted briefly again and the same family members were quickly ushered out and away into the corridor. Almost in the same moment, two men from the mortuary arrived with a long grey bag which they unzipped and took through the gap in the curtain. I heard them moving about around the bed. They were discussing the results of a football match they had seen on the TV the night before and the outrage of their best player being yellow-carded.

"The fucking ref should have been shot for that fucking decision," said one and they both laughed. I let out a pitiful little laugh too as the tears streamed down my face once more. We all have our own ways of coping.

I buried my head under the covers in shame and to avoid Derek's grinning face. As he did most mornings, he was staring vacantly at me as he pulled down his pyjama bottoms and began his usual plaintive call for help.

Chapter 5

At last I was due to go home. Grace was coming in later that morning with my clothes and I was looking forward to getting out. The usual morning doctors' rounds had started and I was waiting my turn to be seen and of course to be informed that I was to be discharged.

I had seen a nutritionist who told me to eat lots of whatever I fancied. That made me smile as Grace had been quite clear and indeed insistent that when I came home my diet would change. This meant less red meat, less sugar, less wine – basically, less of everything that I liked and that she considered bad for me. I had lost a lot of weight during my stay in hospital, due solely to the fact that I had been allowed little or no food in between scans and checks and surgery. I looked gaunt but actually I felt well enough.

The usual entourage of medics swished into my ward and headed straight for my bed. I was reading a crime novel. The doctor smiled at me, which was unusual, and asked me how I was enjoying the book. He had never asked me anything like that before. I remember thinking how kind it was of him to enquire although for him it seemed a little out of character.

Then suddenly without warning, the curtains were drawn around me and my surgeon knelt at my side. It was he and I together, alone inside my curtained tent. He held his note book in both hands, reminding me of a priest about to give the last rites.

He told me, "I have the results from the pathologist.

"I'm sorry, I'm afraid it's not good news. The blockage in your colon was caused by a 3cm tumour and it was malignant, classified as Dukes' C1 with your lymph nodes involved…"

I can't remember anything else. From the doctor, from my bed and from the ward, my mind drifted off into a world of sheer unadulterated terror where death suddenly stood in front of me.

Chapter 6

I lay there in my bed. Something had just happened. A piece of news. I had been given some news. I had just been given a diagnosis which was the beginning of a life change for me, for my immediate and extended family and for my friends. The piece of news seemed like the dropping of the first atomic bomb. The blast ruptured my mind.

Though the news came to me verbally, it seemed like a written school report. Must do better. Good in parts but failed in Latin. Devastation. What will my parents say when they read this? What will Grace say when I tell her the news?

The news fell on me and passed through me. The effect was immediate and stunning. I had to find a way to avoid its impact. Perhaps it wasn't true! Perhaps I had misheard. Someone else in another bed in another hospital in another world had been given this news and I had just overheard the casual conversation between two people. I had eavesdropped. It was another surgeon and another patient. What if it were me after all? What was this threat? Was it a fact and what would the outcome be if it were true? What would be the manifestation of this fact?

It was as if a new set of laws had just been passed but I hadn't been prepared for them, hadn't been told that they had even been written, let alone had just been adopted, unleashed, made public and now were to be enforced.

Yet after I was told, after I phoned Grace and told her and asked her to come in straightaway, and after the medics had gone, there was more strangeness. I was carrying on as before but the wires were crossed just a little maybe, just enough to allow me to continue to function and yet not be the same anymore. I wasn't suddenly plunged into the dark abyss, no one turned the lights out, and I wasn't drowning in the deepening waters that were now engulfing me. And yet my world felt unreal. The light was no longer natural light. It was as if the whole of my world was illuminated by one continuous blinding phosphorous glow.

I wept uncontrollably; made deep sobbing sounds. It felt as if my body had become porous as tears flooded out of every pore. My fingers, hands, limbs and even my head wouldn't move, couldn't be controlled. I was like a beached whale, incapable of moving anywhere.

On hearing the news I wanted to tell people. It felt instinctive. Once I heard the news it could not be rescinded. Nurses came and went. I was counselled. I was looked at with pity and a smile. Others kept away. Perhaps I had an incurable disease that they too would catch if they came too close. So they stayed away. Not too close. The man in the next bed looked at me and then closed his eyes and turned away. Maybe he had already caught the same disease and had already died.

I don't remember many of the other patients being around me, though nurses and visitors stared; they couldn't keep their eyes off me. Cancer and death are so selfish, I thought. I didn't know the protocols and it took me a little while to learn them. Should I chat maybe, or smile? *What have you got? Are you going to live?* And yet compassion was configured over and over again in thin smiles and watery, sad eyes.

I could have been anywhere at any time. Time seemed to be irrelevant then as the length of a day no longer had the measure it possessed before. A day didn't seem a necessary yardstick anymore, nor that morning, nor hours. So many experiences were suddenly all crammed together into a miniscule timeframe that a new timeframe had been created, weird and elastic with no rules. I was no longer living in a real world. In that hospital bed I was sliding down a vertiginous crevasse at a dangerous speed and heading nowhere but oblivion.

In retrospect my aim was simply not to die.

Grace arrived. I called to her. She came and sat with me. I touched her and spoke her name through quivering lips. She was with me and we were together. She was then and still is the most important person in my life. Grace has saved me many times from the abyss, the deepening waters and the darkest of days. We were together, my wife and I. What to tell the children? I remember saying that we would all be changed by this, but without any knowledge of the outcome, just the potential of a negative one.

I wanted to go home, to leave that terrible news room, to seek comfort in familiar surroundings with my loving family, the warm cocoon of my life; clean, complete and safe. It was early days but we needed to prepare, we had to talk about this and make plans for whatever was going to come. I don't remember the journey home, just the arriving.

I had to tell the children. They were summoned and I suppose they suspected they were going to hear the worst. They arrived and we sat together in the lounge. The tears already flowed as I began to explain my situation and its undoubted, definitely positive, outcome, albeit my explanation was peppered with potential negative possibilities. They listened and cried a little and did what I expected of my girls. They told me they would be there for me and as a family we would face the future together, whatever was in store for us. But really, none of us knew what was going to happen.

I loved them then and I love them even more now. Our family unit would stand. This alone wouldn't necessarily be enough to save us, but it was going to give me the strength to continue. Our decision was joint and tacit and was to help save me. Grace and I talked about countless things and kept talking and sometimes crying. We arrived at a point where we could agree to move on and we did.

Chapter 7

I received a letter confirming my appointment to see my surgeon Mr P on Thursday 27 September 2012, at 12.30 pm. The letter confirmed my diagnosis: the blockage in my colon had been caused by a 3cm tumour, graded as Dukes' C1. This meant that some lymph nodes, outside the gut, had also been invaded, but it wasn't known how serious this was. The CT scan showed that the tumour had been removed successfully and also that my liver was clear.

I was to have many more CT scans; a PET scan would also be needed to check the whole of my body; in addition I was to have a colonoscopy to check the rest of the colon, but that would be later.

As for treatment, a course of chemotherapy would be required even though the tumour had been removed. This would start four to six weeks later. I would have eight cycles of treatment, one every three weeks, consisting of an infusion of drugs that would last two hours, with tablets for the next two weeks and a rest for the third week before the next cycle started.

Blood tests between each cycle would determine whether the next cycle could start on time. Whatever that meant.

Grace stepped into *support mode* straight away. She was and is an amazing woman, partner and supporter. A flu jab was organised for me, multivitamins bought, supplements purchased – olive leaf and milk thistle. A list of questions for Mr P was drawn up and battle commenced.

The meeting with Mr P was matter-of-fact. I don't remember too many of the details as I floated in and out of listening mode. Grace made notes.

The colon perforation and tumour had been masked by an abscess. It was a T4 perforation. The microscopic examination had shown that between two and 13 lymph nodes had signs of tumour growth, but that no affected cells had been left behind when the tumour was removed. Again, Mr P stated that my liver was clear.

My surgeon arranged for me to have a second scan within the next two weeks and explained that although the liver was clear it was possible that some cancer cells could appear elsewhere, although this was unlikely. I was prescribed loperamide to "slow the bowel movements down", in his words.

Well I sure as hell needed that!

I was also to see an oncologist and a meeting was set up with her, Dr J, at the Stoke Mandeville cancer clinic in October. I would need four to six weeks to get over all the surgery, allow the wounds to heal, for my overall strength to return and to put some weight on. I was a bag of bones. Most people who came to see me thought I must be already dead.

The risk of infection due to the chemotherapy treatment was the most worrying aspect of all this for me. I could quite easily become neutropenic – suffering from reduced levels of white blood cells and thus a weakened immune system – and that would mean hospitalisation at best. If not treated, possible life-threatening infections would do what the tumour, so far, had failed to do. The thought of A&E again, especially at my local hospital, sent shivers down my bony back.

I was given a booklet as well as being told verbally of the many down-sides of chemotherapy treatment that would or might affect me. Some of these problems could be medicated for – like nausea, vomiting and diarrhoea – while others, like chapped and cracked hands and feet, and pins and needles, could be tackled with E45 cream. Wearing gloves turned out to be the most beneficial protection for my hands, especially around the house. Grace and I both suspected that I would go bald as my hair was falling out in clumps, but I was told that this might not happen, though then again it might. At best I should expect my hair to "thin out". Another wonderful side effect to look forward to was possible choking, but that could be eased by taking warm drinks.

Mmm… in my mental fog I was confused anyway, but by now I was totally lost.

Tiredness was to become the first problem I experienced, while peripheral neuropathy – sensitivity and pain in my hands and feet – became a more serious issue later. Overall, neuropathy was the worst side effect of the chemotherapy and remains with me today.

By the end of the meeting with Mr P, I was not only confused but now frightened, as was my whole family. I desperately needed to understand how the treatment was to be planned and conducted as well as what side effects would become prevalent. I sank into a dark place and cried. I wanted to know what options I had, if any. The shock still hadn't worn off and my life had become suspended, in a place where it remained for the next two years. The discussions and decisions that took place during my initial consultation with my specialist were to be crucial to my future.

I learnt a lot. I learnt that I was mortal. I thought I knew this before but it was at this point that I first fully realised that although I had heard it said many times, only now did I understand it.

Our lives suddenly slowed down as if in a fog above and below us, treacle. One moment just followed another without much purpose at this time. This threat had dual aspects, one that was current, tangible, painful and real; the other was more obscure, the outcome of the threat not known. Hopefully everything would be all right. After all, the surgeon had specified that the tumour was gone, the liver was intact and other possible cancer cells would be annihilated by the chemo treatment. The first was fact and immediate and now. The second was possible but distant, to be determined somewhere in the fog.

I was in a new physical state. It had to be explained to me because it was new, unexpected and bespoke and yet I didn't really feel any different at that time, apart from suffering the after-effects of the surgery. Where was this deadly cancer? I didn't know. Is that why I felt terrifyingly casual about the whole thing or was it the fog or the halting treacle that made us both feel like this?

We carried on with our life, sometimes just as before. We weren't suddenly plunged into darkness. It was still daylight and yet on my shoulder sat a new unnatural light. A shadow, a shade of light that wasn't quite as illuminating, a diffused daylight. These were the first days and I didn't realise just how many days there were going to be like this.

So we started to speak together and communicate to others – friends and family. Grace was my conduit. We wanted to tell people, we needed to tell people and share the information. Grace needed to share the burden of what had happened, what might happen and what we both feared might happen. People spoke and listened and they were always on hand – well most of them anyway. Some people disappeared for reasons unknown. We all deal with frightening issues in different ways, but it did disappoint me. There was a strange quality to our lives. It felt distant and unreal. Sometimes I felt that I was drowning, only to be saved as Grace comforted me with words of hope. Many hours seemed to pass without conscious thoughts, just extending the day into night. At dusk most evenings a smoky wall would descend. I was living in a cell with people coming and going and things happening around me and yet I wasn't really aware of any of it.

Sitting in our lounge with the log burner going; wrapped up in a blanket and comfortable clothes, T-shirts and jogging pants, big jumpers and warm socks. It was bloody autumn, not winter yet and still I felt cold. I called these clothes my "sloppy joes", easy to wear, comfortable. In them I looked like a worn-out old man.

We kept people informed. Well, Grace did mainly. We remembered to contact most people anyway. I didn't want to make new friends. It would have felt fraudulent somehow. The people were family, friends. Personal and some professional. People we loved and had strong bonds with and some we knew a little less, close and near.

There was the constant retelling of the same story until it began to be overwhelming, boring or draining to the point where my spirit became empty. Cancer is a hard thing to talk about and I think it must be even harder to hear, but I didn't have much else to talk about at the time. It was all-consuming so I began to sound dull and boring. People wanted the same details, well they did to a point: a sudden A&E emergency... hospital... scans... surgery... more surgery... a tumour... cancer treatment... then what? Uncertainty. It will be alright. Don't worry.

We didn't want to over-burden our friends with too much detail. They would listen but sometimes they didn't seem to hear, didn't get past the word "cancer". Images would rise up of demons and death. I could see their minds whirring and their listening powers diminish as the fear seeped in.

Glad it's not me. Sorry it's you, but so glad it's not me. I could hear the silent thoughts followed by the slightly open mouth and blank stare, furrowed brow and maybe an uncomfortable squirm. They had been called to witness. We didn't want to give people the wrong idea or information but we didn't really know what the "idea" was. It was an ugly mess made of accurate data mixed with an estimated projection of measured hope. We had statistics and booklets and data from the internet and yet I found myself on that sofa looking deep into the flickering flames of the log fire and seeing my world get darker and darker at times, until I found myself buried in a black hole of utter despair with tears running down my face and dripping off my chin onto my sloppy joes.

I found a new closeness with some friends. Nick visited me in the A&E bed during my two-night stay there before the tumour was found. Dr Ron bore gifts of magazines and other prezzies. Sisters and daughters came of course. But some family members stayed away and some haven't visited to this day. There were no rehearsals for these responses. Again, Grace did most of the communicating which left me to rest and brood at the same time. Over and over we got so many offers of help and love, which were very precious and gratefully received, but our story had become public knowledge now. Our position was noted. Our situation had been heard and at each response a true friend was activated. Our message had a single note that was now becoming a chord and would turn into our psalm.

The family was stressed. I was stressed. The facts were still a little sparse. I had undergone the surgery and the tumour was out. Yet the treatment still hadn't started. Probably chemotherapy, followed by radiotherapy. That's just how it goes, the surgeon told us. The stoma would most probably be reversed in six months' time, even though I had lost a third of my colon. Monitoring would follow, maybe for years.

As a treat and to get me out of the house, Grace planned an evening at the theatre. I was strong enough but still underweight and sitting on my bony bottom on a theatre seat for a couple of hours wasn't my idea of a comfortable evening's entertainment, despite the promise of a strawberry and chocolate ice cream at the interval. As I settled into my seat, Grace spied old neighbours of ours whom we hadn't seen for several years. They rushed over to say hello, smiling, but as Grace informed them about our new "situation", I watched the husband's face change. The smile disappeared as he turned to look at me. His gaze disturbed me as a blank stare set in his eyes and froze his face. He stared and stared at me. Perhaps I wasn't even there. Perhaps he was looking straight through me as the dreaded cancer word sank deeper into his mind. They turned and took their seats and I haven't seen them since.

Chapter 8

I met with my oncologist Dr J for the first time on 23 October 2012, at the Stoke Mandeville cancer clinic. She was tall and slim with an open, friendly face and bright, inquisitive eyes that seemed to sparkle when she smiled. It was a wonderfully big, welcoming smile. Empathy seemed to flow out of her and I felt straightaway that I would like her, believe in her and above all trust her.

Her first words to me as she scanned the now thick pile of "my" notes that she had on her desk were, "My word, but you have been through the wars."

"Yes, I have," I replied and followed it with, "and I ask you for only one thing. The truth. Always tell me the truth."

She promised me that she would do that and, to this day, I know she always has.

Dr J's mind obviously worked at twice the speed of most people's, including Grace's and mine. She spoke quickly and with confidence to summarise our situation, my condition and the treatment I would be receiving, but before that she invited me to read through the notes she had clasped in her hands. My notes.

The notes from my surgeon Mr P and his team. Grace and I had been suspicious about the reasons for my second operation because we had been given conflicting information; we were still very unclear as to what had really happened. Yet here was Dr J offering to explain to me the reasons for that operation, wanting to tell me the truth from Day One, wanting me to understand clearly what was written in the medical file.

My oncologist always interested me. It's true that it took me a while to get used to her. I wasn't sure why she never seemed to be alarmed at our conversations or findings, but that was before we started to understand about alarming outcomes. I was always glad when we saw Dr J. She was my *fait accompli* – here is your cancer and here is your cancer doctor – but she always made me feel better just by seeing her and being with her. Dr J was always our bearer of tidings, good and sometimes bad, and she was always in control of the rich implications of my situation and presented them to me with authority and yet with a soothing voice.

She analysed the data and would explain them to me quickly and factually. The facts continued to emerge until they ran out and at that point she stopped talking. Dr J always pictured what my cancer was doing and when it was misbehaving. She had, no doubt, pictured conditions like mine many times before in many patients and had the ability to plot them carefully in her head. Although she always talked quickly and was always behind with her patients, she knew not to describe everything at once but to compress our discussions. She was constantly working against the clock as there were always so many patients to be seen, though this was a pressure of which I was hardly aware due to her communication skills and organisational efficacy.

Dr J was serious when that was required and she always made sure she did things right. Yet we found that we could make each other laugh. Doctor and patient were in some ways on a similar level. I felt she understood my disease scientifically, acted with integrity, could identify my progress by looking at me (and Grace behind my back) and was vigilant at dealing with my condition. In the clinic, when I found myself vividly relating an event – a recent trip to India perhaps, or a story involving one of our girls – I would feel that there was pleasure in it for the two of us. Her lovely smiling eyes would widen with laughter as she looked at Grace and me, but then narrowed again as she leaned in to examine my notes

It became very apparent in that consultation that, during my first operation, a drainage tube had been accidently inserted into my intestine instead of my abdomen wall, which not only did not drain the fluid build-up in my abdomen cavity but was now infecting the whole area.

I can't remember much more about that conversation as a red mist was not only colouring my vision but also helping me to lose my hearing. The anger that took hold of me was immense. Dr J became aware of my rage and carefully and sensibly steered me away from drastic action. I was already fantasising about returning home to pick up my red-tipped axe! She explained that I would need to take up the issue with my surgeon as she had only one role, one intention and one focus – to prescribe and manage my future treatment.

The pathology report stated that my cancer had extended beyond my colon to "involve" the lymph nodes outside and, as there could be many loose cancer cells floating menacingly around my pelvic area, Dr J prescribed treatment by radiotherapy initially, followed by chemotherapy. Recent CT scans of my chest and a full-body MRI scan had come back "clear and normal", so I was to be put on a five-week radiotherapy course. In practice, this would consist of doses of 25 radiation "fractions" being zapped into me. A fraction is a small dose of radiation, the dose being divided thus in order to allow healthy cells to recover between treatments. The fractions were to be delivered externally from a large machine and each would take a few minutes. There would be 25 fractions for five consecutive days over five weeks. There would be no treatment over the weekends. This adjuvant radiotherapy is really just an application of high-energy radiation, like x-rays, designed to destroy any remaining cancer cells without destroying me. I was told it wouldn't make me radioactive or make me glow in the dark, although I quite liked the idea of the latter.

The treatment would begin at the cancer clinic in three weeks, Dr J explained, along with a long list of possible negative side effects, the first being death! After radiotherapy I was to have eight cycles of two chemotherapy drugs designed for my condition, capecitabine and oxaliplatin.

Two weeks later I received a copy of a letter that Dr J had sent to my GP. Neither he nor any other GP from the medical centre came to see me then or over the past five years. The letter had also been copied to Mr P.

The letter clearly indicated my diagnosis: *Rectal adenocarcinoma pT4 N2/13 on 10 September 2012. Low Hartman's procedure and a right hemicolectomy.*

The letter went on to inform my GP that I had made an excellent post-operative recovery (by this she meant physically, not necessarily mentally) and my performance status was zero (meaning that I was basically OK). I had gained weight and I was managing my stoma well.

The letter went on to say:

I discussed the intra-operative and pathology findings – recommending pelvic chemo-radiotherapy due to the tumour perforations. This will involve 25 fractions of radiotherapy given daily on weekdays with oral capecitabine chemotherapy on the days of radiotherapy. I have been through the acute and late toxicity of chemo-radiotherapy including the risk of death from infections, blood clots and heart problems. Having radiotherapy to the pelvis may make subsequent reversal of his stoma more difficult if there is scarring. Adjuvant chemotherapy will take place subsequent to radiotherapy.

I was summoned to the surgery to receive, complete and sign a statement of (lack of) fitness to work, effectively signing me off for six months. But I still had my consultancy business to run. My study at home was an ideal place for this. My plan was to continue developing a programme with a big global client and get to India the following year if possible.

Not fit to work? Pah!

Once I had regained sufficient weight, the radiotherapy treatment started on 21 November 2012 at the Churchill Hospital in Oxford, and was to be completed the day after Boxing Day, followed by an appointment with Dr J in early January 2013.

Chapter 9

Receiving radiotherapy treatment inside a linear accelerator takes only five minutes, but add on parking in any of the hospital car parks that could take 20 minutes, plus the travel to the Churchill Hospital and back, the preparation time, the tardiness of previous patients and treatment issues and each session took at least half a day. Grace came with me every time.

Now, I am not an advocate of tattoos. I am not against other people having them and I am sure many female football supporters find the inked skin of top-rated players attractive, but I don't like tattoos and I especially don't like them on me.

Yet I now have three! This strange circumstance came about because of the radiotherapy. In order to ensure that I was always placed in exactly the same position to be "zapped" in the accelerator, I had to have three tiny stars tattooed onto me. Lasers used these spots to align me exactly to the x-rays. I had one star tattooed on the small of my back and two more, one on each hip. Cool or what? I have often offered to show people my "tats", but when they realise where they are located and that they are virtually impossible to detect without a magnifying glass, they generally lose interest.

The treatment swallowed up all of our pre-Christmas preparations that year. Most of the celebrations passed us by as we made the daily pilgrimage to the Churchill Hospital. Weekends provided the only respite and I took the time to rest. Despite the constant routine, I can say that the experience at that hospital lifted me up. Later, I addressed a conference of pharmacists with a patient's perspective on coping with the side effects of post-chemotherapy drugs along with the other essentials: good nursing, good oncologists, right drugs, caring family and friends. I told the pharmacists that the Churchill provided that kind of environment in which treatment is offered.

The moment I arrived at the Churchill, a new building with a large, light and open atrium, wide, well-lit and bright corridors hung with photographs and pictures, a large reception area and relaxed staff who were focused, capable and apparently happy, I was *made to feel better*. The wonderful and effective radiographers and radiotherapists were always busy and were obviously hard working, but they didn't appear to be suffering under the usual NHS stress. The after-care nurses ensured my personal details were always up to date, my questions always answered and my physical needs met. It made me realise just how important the environmental impacts were on helping patients recover. The treatment room surroundings, hospitals, nurses and doctors I had encountered all played a positive part in how I was coping with cancer.

I was taking capecitabine twice a day in 1,650mg doses. I had to use mouth wash to keep the ulcers away and metoclopramide

49

to stop me vomiting. I had a blood test every Friday and would wait anxiously over the weekend, hoping the results were good, that my haemoglobin levels and white blood cell levels were high. My radiotherapy treatment went well. Although I had been informed about the avalanche of possible side effects, I wasn't prepared for the peripheral neuropathy which was to become continuous across the treatment and beyond, but initially I found it could be controlled with daily applications of an aqueous cream.

The radiographers and I laughed and shared banal conversations as I undressed to lie face down on the trolley with my bare bum in the air, before the lasers homed in on my tattoos to line me up. The technicians occasionally had to manhandle me into position by slapping either buttock – gently I might add – until the laser beam guidance system was aligned. I do remember a new female radiographer from New Zealand, who had started at the Churchill just that week, getting rather exasperated with me, as alignment was eluding her and she was having to manipulate me more than she would have liked. Before she realised what she had said, she accused me of moving about so much that it provoked her into slapping me a bit too hard. The others laughed and asked if I enjoyed it, just as the electronic trolley slipped me into the body of the radiotherapy machine, ready to be given my 45Gy Rx dose, which means my prescription was for 45 grays of radiation.

During this time I was feeling quite fit, energised as much by the environment and staff at the Churchill as by having my family and close friends around me and the treatment going well. The expected negative side effects were by no means as bad as they could have been, even though some were beginning to take hold.

I put on more weight, as I needed to. I felt better within myself mentally as well as physically. I liked to eat and it annoyed Grace that the nutritionists and dieticians told me I could eat whatever I wanted. I was greedy for butter and cream. Sauces and puddings and ice cream and milk shakes were back on the menu. Large portions became my mantra. I drew up a new anti-diet sheet that read, *fried food, 12-inch diameter plates, pile it high and don't worry if it slides over the edge, please come back for seconds.* Sometimes I did need to mention the words "cancer treatment" to get my second helping though.

People would come up to me knowing that I had been diagnosed with cancer and say, "But you look so well." This sometimes made me laugh but often I would have to ask them why they said that. What did they want me to look like? What did they *expect* me to look like? Did I need to look thin, pale and grey just so that it would confirm their expectations of what cancer must do to you? Did my armpits have to look like white caverns in their sockets, my eyes sunken into my skull, my head shaven before I fitted the bill?

Every time this happened, I remember whispering to myself, *I will win, I will beat this. Together with my family and my true friends we will triumph together.*

Chapter 10

To have completed five weeks of the daily slog into Oxford for the radiotherapy treatment was indeed a relief. I had a week before we were due to see Dr J, my oncologist, again, five days before my 60th birthday.

Grace made sure that my birthday was the best that could be arranged under the circumstances. Having lots of people around me didn't seem like a great idea, not so soon after intensive radiotherapy treatment and not forgetting my aim of remaining well enough to start chemotherapy on time. I found it difficult to focus on anything but what was to come. So in the end we asked the girls round for a quiet dinner at home. It was wonderful just to have them with me. It always has been. I love them so very dearly.

I was to start the eight cycles of oxaliplatin and capecitabine chemotherapy on 15 January 2013, but this treatment was delayed until I had yet more blood tests. Dr J was confident that the chemotherapy was going to be a *mopping up exercise*, so we were confident too. We had to be, as the only alternative was too frightening to consider, too opaque to see beyond.

We trusted, but we didn't know.

My father, being exactly 30 years older than me, was dealing with old age. He was 90 years old three days earlier and, like me, celebrated his birthday with the help of all his children and, in his case, grandchildren. We all travelled up to see him in Harrogate, North Yorkshire, but he wasn't well due to a chest infection and had fallen over again, so was in hospital. I didn't visit him in hospital as Grace, thoughtful as ever, was concerned that I might pick up an infection from the ward or even from my father. Instead I sat in the car in the car park for what seemed an age, reading a book on Roman history by Mary Beard.

While waiting in the car park with my iPhone, Grace sent photos and a short video of my father waving to me, wishing me happy birthday. I am sure he must have wondered why I wasn't there in person. I hadn't told him that I had cancer. I don't know why. I didn't want to upset or worry him I suppose. What would have been the purpose of him knowing? What would he have been able to do to help? He died a couple of weeks later, still not knowing. I thought it was for the best. He knew that I was in hospital the previous year and that I had several operations, but beyond that, as he never asked me why, I didn't tell him the full extent of my condition. Maybe he knew, but he never asked me. Maybe I should have told him, maybe not.

After the blood tests, treatment started at the Stoke Mandeville cancer clinic on 22 January at 11.00 am. I didn't ever attend these sessions alone. Grace always came with me for my treatment and although she would leave me for the two-to-three-hour duration, she would always be there to pick me up, drive me home and help with the side-effect issues and the mental upset that occurred during every cycle. Grace was my reason for living. She was always my rock. Without her I don't think I would be writing this today. I loved her always, but this was a test that drew us closer together than ever before, in all the 42 years we had so far been together.

It was my first day of treatment back at my local hospital. I sat in the waiting area. I knew more or less what I had to go through. I had to see Dr J first, then be weighed, then meet a stoma nurse in case I had any issues, or questions, or problems to discuss. I felt suddenly paralysed with depression. The hospital clinic was a new building, as the Churchill was, but here the receptionists always seemed to have the incorrect booking dates. The queue at reception was long, the lack of seating frustrating and the small and inadequate waiting area, used by both cancer patients and haematology patients, claustrophobic and dark. Even the post-Christmas look was tainted by the space on the wall where a plaque celebrating the shamed former friend of the hospital, Jimmy Savile, had once hung but had now been not-so-discreetly removed.

The waiting area was over-crowded. An elderly couple sat across from us. The wife was very thin and frail. She raised her eyes to look at me and with a faint smile closed them again and sighed deeply. I felt the prickle start at the back of my eyes, not knowing if the welling tears were for her or for me.

And so it began.

I found myself in one of three rather cramped rooms, each of which had several large, comfortable, plastic-coated armchairs – easier to clean the blood off, as I was later to learn. So many chairs and yet never enough for the patients *and* guests. These rooms were for patients to be comfortable, not private. A guest could sit with you. The nursing staff were friendly and helpful. They were sometimes rushed but in the main they managed with systematic precision. I was settled down for the two or three hours the treatment was going to take.

Finding veins to plug into was always an interesting start. I got used to collapsed veins and bruised arms and sometimes painful insertions, but it was all part of the process, something we all went through while we sat facing others having similar treatment. Whichever arm was to be attacked was rested on a crisp white pillow. Microwaved bags of barley were used to prepare my arm, keeping it warm and allowing the major veins to swell in preparation for needles.

There were prints of flowers on the walls, pointless, dull and old. The heating was turned up high to keep us warm. Trolleys and frames and buckets for "sharps" added to the clutter. The lighting was fierce, bright fluorescent strips on polystyrene tiles and the walls painted with washable gloss. I was nervous, not frightened, just uncomfortably nervous.

I was to be given oxaliplatin, a drug used when there has been confirmation that the bowel cancer has spread locally into the lymph nodes. This was given as an infusion in conjunction with capecitabine. First though, I had a saline solution flush followed by 6mg of dexamethasone in a 0.9-percent saline solution, followed by the oxaliplatin over two hours and finally a glucose intravenous flush before I could escape. I watched the slow intravenous (IV) infusion dripping from a transparent bag suspended from a bracket above me, dripping and running through the tube and into my vein. I was to receive these chemicals every two or three weeks, depending on my physical condition and the side effects of the drugs. In my case these were nausea, sometimes followed by vomiting and always diarrhoea.

Every evening after that treatment I had to take capecitabine and an anti-emetic, ondansetron, to stop me throwing up. A day later I also took a general steroid, used as another anti-emetic, dexamethasone.

And so it continued. The same routine every time.

I had the occasional nose bleed, sore gums and some bruising, but generally I got by without too much discomfort. The main issue for me, caused by the oxaliplatin, was severe peripheral neuropathy. It started from the very beginning, only in my fingers to start with, but once I got home it migrated to my left arm and although milder, also to my throat and feet. Once it caused me to have a sneezing fit over a bag of chocolate Minstrels – not a pretty sight.

Reaching into the fridge once to get some milk, I couldn't bear to touch the cold carton and dropped it on the floor where it broke. I was shocked. It was as if an electric current had shot up my arm. I burst into tears, sat down and cried. The numbness and tingling in my fingers was because the nerves had been damaged by the drugs. The effect was tolerable during normal day-to-day activity but to be unable to hold cold things, or even put my hand in the fridge, was painful. As it got worse, I couldn't touch anything made of steel, like the microwave oven, dishwasher or our range cooker.

The feeling of peripheral neuropathy was like shards of ice being jabbed into my arm whilst at the same time it was being thrust into a bucket of ice just enough that the pain remained without it going numb. The same would happen on my tongue if I tried to eat ice cream. It was like eating small pieces of frozen glass.

I think Grace considered my complaints just a smart way of getting out of doing chores around the house. To allay her suspicions I began wearing gloves to get things out of the fridge and had to wrap up more, especially as it was still winter. The symptoms got worse and then spread to my toes and feet, Although the drugs that I take now help, my toes still hurt to this day.

I came home after that first cycle of treatment totally exhausted, upset and depressed. I had to take capsules of capecitabine orally, twice a day for 14 days, followed by a seven-day break, until my next cycle of treatment was due. Taking that cycle would be dependent on the blood test results that would indicate whether I was fit enough for more treatment. I always looked forward to those seven days, but not the blood tests that would follow, or rather their results.

The greatest fear and threat was the increased risk of infection and neutropenic sepsis. Infection at any time during my treatment could have a major effect, not only on my level of tolerance of the treatment and retarding my recovery, but if my white-cell count dropped and I had a serious infection then it could kill me. It was the one thing that was to haunt me through the whole of my treatment. I was to receive a couple of serious scares. On one occasion I was suddenly struck by a severe fever caused by an infection linked to the low levels of neutrophil white cells in my blood. This landed me back in the now-familiar local A&E department where I spent several hours waiting to be seen before I could be treated. When my case eventually came up it was judged a medical emergency and I was hooked up to an antibiotic IV line just in time. This saved me.

After this I had to take my blood pressure regularly and my temperature daily. The slightest increase in temperature always sent us into stress and panic mode.

Chapter 11

After my first cycle of chemotherapy, I would sit quietly at home most days. No one disturbed me. Grace was constantly there to keep me warm, fed and generally looked after. We would talk quietly. I wanted to run away, catch a plane and hide somewhere. I didn't want to go back to the clinic and see *those people*. I meant the other patients. They all had cancer for goodness' sake. Women with head scarves and no eyebrows. Old men with grey-yellow complexions. Companions with sad faces and red, sore eyes from too many tears. Happy bloody nurses busy caring and volunteers serving tea and coffee and sandwiches and yoghurts from the hospital canteen at lunch times.

There were many times when I couldn't initiate a conversation. Usually Grace would begin to speak and I would join in. I developed the habit of waiting to be involved in conversation, waiting to have a reason to talk, even though sometimes I thought I wasn't ready. I was often sad but in a new way. I wondered if I would ever be sad again in a normal way. Was this just a puzzle that I had to solve? The dark place would creep up on me and the demon on my left shoulder would appear just to remind me.

Home comforts were essential, animal comforts – warmth, being at ease, good food. Also, of course, an immediate, close, loving family, and friends who were amazingly supportive and generous with their time and kindness.

I was mobile enough to know I could run. Because I could, sometimes I thought I would run away and hide and nobody would find me. How easy would it be to catch a plane to Switzerland, I wondered? Where was that clinic, the one that let you decide the ultimate about your life for yourself? Trust and belief and hope somehow kept me from running away and catching that plane, along with the deep, reciprocated love that I had for my wife and family. I knew I had to believe in the science and the medicines, the hospitals and the clinics. I had to trust my oncologist, my truth teller, my saviour. I decided that belief and trust were the best solution.

I stayed.

We were together, Grace and I. Our three girls were close enough. I wondered whether I would die. How would Grace and the girls cope if I did? They would always be mine, but how would I be able to love them if I wasn't there? The lack of knowledge about loving, that was my constant concern and it would take me into my dark place, the place that was marked with a black cross. If I couldn't love them and they couldn't love me, then what?

I wanted the treatment. Of course I had to stay. I was afraid of what might happen if I left. I would not leave. I would stay and fight and love. I was being given the chance to live and love and I just had to get used to it.

Those January days were short and the slate-grey skies morphed seamlessly from cold late morning light into dark, damp late afternoons. The treatment cycles continued through those cold months. Grace was always my companion, always by my side. Dr J provided expert advice and solutions to actual and potential problems. We went to and from the clinic feeling like nomads, homeless and bodiless. Nurses smiled as they drove needles into my veinless arms. They were only going through the inevitable motions. It was organised and had to be accepted.

Waiting and sitting and explaining and talking and needles and infusions and nausea and increasingly painful hands and arms, and all the time I still had to get used to my stoma. Trying and sometimes failing to manage the constant changing of bags and cleaning and having to be careful about what I ate and when, never knowing if a bag would split or whether I would be able to reach a toilet in time. Putting soiled stoma bags in black plastic bags with all the wet and dry wipes needed to keep me clean. Sealing the black bags to deposit them discreetly in the rubbish bins outside. It was all too embarrassing to discuss with anyone except the specialist stoma nurses and Grace.

The first three cycles of chemotherapy took place as scheduled, but before my fourth cycle was due to take place, I was told I had a problem. The blood tests showed that I was neutropenic – low on neutrophil white blood cells. My count was 1.3 and as the minimum healthy level was 1.5 it meant I couldn't have further treatment. The platelet and total white blood cell levels were also slightly low, so my treatment was postponed for at least 10 days at which point resuming the chemotherapy would depend on whether I was well enough. My treatment programme didn't start again until the end of April. The same thing happened again in May – neutropenia called another halt to my treatment. Obviously I needed to be fit enough for the chemotherapy, but the frustration was killing me! I was getting depressed at not being able to get on with the treatment.

I was determined that none of this was going to stop me from living my life.

All this time I was still working at my consultancy business. A major client wanted me to develop and run a big project in India. It started that March and was due to run for 18 months. I worked from home, where I could develop the necessary programmes and keep track of the contract through meetings with the client's project manager. I went to India three times during this period, despite the issues with travel insurance. I needed to work. I needed to live my life again as much as possible. Working saved me from going mad.

I travelled to India in April to deliver a big training programme for my client's staff, and again in May for some calibration work. Trying to manage these trips in between treatment sessions was an interesting balancing act. Most people thought I was mad even to think about going on such arduous journeys to Asia. What if you're ill? What about insurance? My view was simple. What about dying before I finished the work? I would never forgive myself.

Immersing myself in such a large and challenging consultancy project was exactly what I needed to keep my mind active and focused on anything except what was actually happening to me. I was to travel to India again in August, while in between I worked with an assistant who came for meetings with me regularly to catch up with progress, exchange information and sometimes, when treatment and the demands of work clashed, be relied upon to deliver some of the project himself.

Despite the time difference, I used to phone Grace from my travels regularly so that she knew I was doing well, and I emailed her virtually every day with updates on progress with my work and health. The effects of the treatment, and particularly the peripheral neuropathy, were sometimes an issue, but as the temperature in Bangalore was usually around the forties Celsius, it seemed less painful. On the other hand, due to *India's rich cuisine*, my stoma was a constant issue and I was often caught short or had to make a sudden excuse to work colleagues to disappear from a restaurant table to change my stoma bag.

In April, Dr Ron, one of my most supportive friends, asked me if I would be willing to give a short – 20-minute – paper at a pharmaceutical conference to be held in Edinburgh, Scotland on 8 May. I jumped at the chance. He of course was concerned about my mental state, as the conference organisers wanted me to present an account of my personal journey through coping with the effects of post-chemotherapy drugs.

In Edinburgh I stood on the podium surveying the sea of faces. In the audience were some of Europe's leading pharmacists. I remember clearly the way they looked at me. Total, stunned silence filled the room as I presented my story. They understood the science, the pharmacological facts, and yet the painful, personal aspects of my use of their drugs seemed to stop them in their tracks. They didn't really know how to react to someone standing in front of them with a stoma, still being treated for cancer and explaining the side effects of post-chemotherapy meds in detail.

I was asked few questions until the conference day came to an end. Then several individuals, one with tears in his eyes, told me how brave I was to speak in public; others told me how it had helped them consider working on alternatives to some drugs and treatments. A psychologist wanted to know more about my thoughts on a holistic approach that not only involved the mental and physical importance of treatment, but also the environmental one.

Travelling home, I decided I was proud of what I had said and pleased that I had spoken. I felt good about myself and my future.

Apart from the conference and my work in India, I had nothing to do but wait. Occasionally, Grace would take me out for a drive or to do some shopping. We would have tea and cakes somewhere. It was good to get out of the house but I am not sure we would have spent so much time in cafés with a pot of Darjeeling and two toasted tea cakes if I had been in treatment still. But it kept my spirits up and, as there was no one there to stop us, I felt we were being a pair of mavericks. We would lean against each other and hold hands as we did in the cancer clinic, on those green chairs in the reception area waiting to see Dr J.

I didn't see Dr J again until early June, just after my fifth treatment cycle, due to the cancellations caused by my low blood counts. The oxaliplatin dose was reduced to 80 percent to help me tolerate it better. Grace came with me as usual, and sat slightly behind me. I couldn't see her face and reactions. Even more annoyingly, Dr J would always look at her over my shoulder, seeking confirmation of my situation, health, mental state and coping ability. A stoma nurse sat at my other side and received the same over-my-shoulder looks from Dr J. The glances between Dr J, Grace and the nurse were like visual ping pong, with me the umpire, playing piggy in the middle.

I still had grade 1 peripheral neuropathy, Dr J informed me, as if I needed to be told. Although the discomfort of this wasn't causing me any functional impairment, it was still annoying. The chemotherapy was also causing issues with my stoma although I was beginning to manage things better in that area. My loperamide dosage was increased to help me manage my stoma even more easily. These decisions seemed to be agreed by nods and winks behind my back, ping pong between Dr J, Grace and the stoma nurse.

My next cycle of treatment began in mid-May. At the same time, the state of my neuropathy was to be reviewed and if there was no reduction in the level of pain, the oxaliplatin was going to be stopped. There had been no change, so the treatment was continued after discussions with Dr J. My treatment was interrupted again due to my neutropenia despite the fact that I felt well enough and my performance status was still rated zero, meaning that officially I was fully active and able to carry on activities without restriction.

Despite this rating I was gradually getting more tired and it was beginning to show in everything I did. At least the early summer warmth and long days of glorious, sunlit evenings were making life more tolerable. But the nausea was getting worse and

I vomited after my last treatment, which left me more tired and upset than before. The positive prognosis from Dr J was that *things will get worse before they start to get better* with regard to my neuropathy, by which she meant after my whole treatment was completed. I was to continue with cycles seven and eight, after which I would have another CT scan in September.

More good news: I was to have a consultation with Dr H, a stoma reversal surgeon. One day I might actually be able to get rid of my bag.

Chapter 12

The nursing staff at the Stoke Mandeville cancer clinic by this time had become well known to me. Some were more diligent than others, and some seemed happier in their work than others. One in particular was easily capable of being embarrassed and I seemed to be able to do that on most of my visits. Why she ever became a nurse totally confounded me, except that I couldn't imagine where else her talents might be used. She was very good at pretending not to hear. Her black hair was always just a little distressed and fixed up in either a ponytail or with a complex network of clips. I wondered if she had ever seen herself from behind. She was easily flustered and always dropping things, including medical samples. Finding a vein in my arm to pierce with a needle seemed to completely flummox her. Another nurse of my acquaintance smiled knowingly when I mentioned this to her as she informed me that the one with the black ponytail was actually a sister, not a nurse.

I didn't get to choose which nurse attended to me and mainly it didn't matter as long as "Sister" wasn't around or she was busy being incompetent elsewhere. This dig may sound mean and ungrateful, but when both your arms are already looking remarkably like pin cushions and are bruised and devoid of any un-collapsed veins, the last thing you need is that particular sister heading your way.

There was one person in charge of each shift and they managed the rest of the team, not that they seemed to need managing as everything ran reasonably smoothly. Everything, that is, except for the delivery of drugs. As this was the responsibility of the hospital pharmacy and not the cancer clinic staff, the nurses could not be taken to task for the all-too-frequent times that the drugs failed to arrive on time. One of the people in charge was a lovely, caring, gentle young black man, who spoke often about his family. I discovered he had studied alongside our eldest daughter Emily in the local hospital library as she was completing her doctorate in clinical psychology. He was like the top steward on our chemotherapy cruise ship, where he carried his authority carefully and gently. He was casually efficient. His manner and approach were ingrained in him. He never hurried and he was always in control, managing well and noticing everything. His smile was like an inverted coat hanger and his laugh was infectious. I looked forward to seeing him along with two or three of the other nurses and auxiliary staff. They were my cancer clinic carers and I grew to love, care about and admire them.

Grace would take me to my appointments, give me a newspaper and a pen for the crosswords, my Kindle to read and extra garments in case I wasn't warm enough, as if this was possible in the over-heated sauna atmosphere of the group treatment rooms!

Grace often sat with me for a little while before heading off to take care of a few jobs or do the shopping. Sometimes we didn't talk. There was no need and anyway sometimes we just didn't. There were times to talk, when we had issues, when we had pain, when we had to talk about what was going on in our life, articulating the disaster that had coagulated around us. We had promised to keep people informed and talk to our children. I needed to talk to them as it was me who this was happening to. Being in the clinic for several hours gave me that time to think about what it was I wanted to say, but so often there were too many distractions and all too often many of the other patients seemed to be in a much worse position than I was. My own situation became so diluted in comparison that I sometimes felt fraudulent for even being there.

As expected, a pattern emerged. The treatment rooms became spaces in which routines developed. There were many very ill patients with whom I sat and waited on every visit, some that I had seen before but many that I hadn't and wouldn't see again.

As regulars now, we all knew who was the patient, who were the family or carers and who were the nursing staff. We cancer patients had a secret, silent language. Our disease, the one we all shared, was invisible. There were no apparent symptoms by which anyone could tell what each of us was suffering from, except for some bald heads and bruised arms. This made finding out – gaining knowledge – vitally important. It could be by asking questions of other patients or by subtle detective work. We all knew that we were there for treatment and we could determine, just by seeing the drugs being infused, what treatment each was having and therefore what the probable cancerous cause was of each patient's dilemma. It was like having knowledge passed on from one to another, from eye to eye.

Sometimes, talking seemed appropriate and a sudden explosion of words would pass between two patients. It was something that we all knew we could do but didn't until given the opportunity. That came only when a supporting carer, family member or nurse was no longer present – for example, between treatment periods, during the long boring infusions or when mum went out for a wee or to the hospital shop for a packet of Quavers. The vacuum would be broken, the void traversed. All our information and news, great and terrible, was imparted in that liminal space. The door would be thrown open for a while and we would verbally run round our own little room until the missing person returned and the door was firmly shut again. But we knew, we had spoken and we understood that the other patient too had the same fear, the same despair, and the same hope.

The camaraderie of the chemo bays was often strangely uplifting, although there were also times of stress and trauma. There was the man who needed a blood transfusion who got more agitated as the nurses fussed around him. His wife stood stationary with sad eyes and a wan smile. I caught her gaze, she smiled a little more and I smiled back. People would get on other people's nerves. Some women discussed their head scarves. The styles and patterns seemed to be the main talking points. A middle-aged man with long, grey hair in a ponytail and leathery, sun-tanned skin sat opposite me, muttering while his partner sat next to him silently disapproving of me writing emails on my iPad.

Everyone came prepared with things like newspapers, food, knitting or puzzle books. People shuffled in and people shuffled out, promenading backwards and forwards to the toilets, dragging their infusion bags on the wheelie coat-hangers as they navigated their way around everyone else sitting in their different-coloured, plastic super armchairs. Patients who had early appointments could choose their chair and claim their own personal preferred position to watch others, have easy access to the nurses and get their tea and biscuits first. Long-standing patients knew well in advance where the best armchairs were and appeared confident in their superior knowledge of the way things happened.

I always tried not to make any fuss and not to show discomfort or annoyance at the tardiness of the drugs being delivered. Sometimes, due to pressure on the hospital pharmacy, our drugs weren't prepared in time for our treatment; we just had to wait. The drugs – the cytotoxics – would arrive on a trolley in thrice-checked, light-resistant, transparent, sealed, plastic bags. I would be asked my name and age and told the names of the toxins I was about to receive. That was the approved, methodical process. But when the medicines arrived late, the procedure was completed in a bit more of a flurry. Late drugs always put everything else behind; you weren't in control.

I was never in control anyway. What could I have done? Sometimes, when my infusion finished and the machine bleeped and bleeped and continued to bleep, trying to catch the attention of the busy nurses was neither possible nor sensible. They were always worked off their feet, always rushing to deal with the next bleeping machine or the next saline flush. Occasionally the intricate and micro workings and tubes of the infusion machines and their drip-feed systems would suddenly stop – they would clog up or just stop functioning for a second or two. The chemo bays were always short of at least one staff member which helped extend the delays still further. People would sit quietly, looking tired and drained and just wait, while others would complain or mutter incoherently without purpose. Those times were the worst times and the most stressful for me as all I could do was watch a situation I was unable to influence, though it was my instinct to try. However, I felt positive that the drugs I was being given were going to make me better so I was always optimistic about my visits to the clinic.

A small, rather fragile-looking old lady had been coming to the clinic for several years. Her reliance on her chemo treatment was obvious in the way she looked at me on the occasions that our appointment times coincided. She was always greeted in the same way. *My, you look lovely today. Had your hair done?* The lady was always beautifully turned out in her tweeds or long dresses and polished court shoes. "I must get home in time for my tea," she would say, looking concerned about the time and expecting her treatment to be delayed as it often was. She looked frayed and nervous as if she were in the customs queue at an airport. I watched as they prepared her. "How's your line? I said, *how's your PICC line?* Your *line?*" She wasn't deaf and she knew the procedure, but part of her was standing in that customs queue, waiting to be called, passport in hand, hoping she would get through without being stopped.

We did the crossword together once. She would give me the clue and I would desperately try and think of a possible answer. Sometimes it was a little difficult as she either didn't tell me how many letters the word should have, or would tell me the wrong number of letters, only to correct herself after five minutes of my providing totally wrong and irrelevant answers. On one occasion, she snapped down her newspaper, stared at me through her silver spectacles with piercing brown eyes and scolded me for suggesting what she quite vehemently considered a ridiculous answer. Three down. *Health worker doctor insured to accommodate firm.* Eight and five letters. I was never sure though if the numbers of letters were right.

Sometimes someone would sit in a corner and stare at me. I would try to avoid their gaze but once or twice I would give them a smile and nod in acknowledgement. On one such occasion, a middle-aged lady stared with bright-eyed interest, like an entomologist looking at a cockroach, and then suddenly closed her eyes and drifted off for a while, head slipping onto her chest. Moments later she pulled herself upright with a snort and continued to stare at me again. She was crisply dressed, but each time she fell asleep she slipped a little lower in her pink plastic armchair and her head scarf slipped at the same time a little further over her forehead, until ultimately it ended up over her eyes as her legs splayed out, her dress rode a little too high above her knees and her machine bleeped loudly, desperately trying to wake her.

There was one session that I found very stressful at the time and even now. A slim, pretty young woman was having her infusion right opposite me. A couple of metres separated us. Her bleach-blonde, rather rotund, mother next to her was reading *OK!* magazine. The young woman had spiky black hair, which I identified as recent re-growth since her last chemo treatment. She seemed happy enough and smiled a lot at me and everyone else around her. The nurses seemed to know her well and engaged with her easily and often. They talked light-heartedly about the lovely warm weather and a recent shopping spree she had been on. She made me feel good and I felt glad that she was happy and positive about her treatment, but I was waiting for the door of opportunity to be thrown open to allow us to have the unspoken conversation that I wanted.

Our chance came when her mother went to the loo. As soon as the toilet door closed, ours opened. She was only 23 and yet had two children, two boys: one five and one three years old. One was helpful and supportive, the other a handful and disruptive. She had been treated for Hodgkin's lymphoma on and off for several years and her boys were her life, her future, her reason for still being here. We exchanged our stories and discussed our hopes and future goals. Her goal, she gleefully explained to me, was to see her boys enjoy Christmas that year.

The door of the toilet swung open and our window of opportunity slammed shut. Her mother, having heard part of our conversation, seemed annoyed and explained to me, quite forcefully, that her daughter's goal was to see the boys' birthdays, one in March the following year and the other two months later.

The young woman just smiled. She looked at me through saddening eyes, wiping away the tear that spilled down her cheek. I fought back the sudden pain that was now scorching the back of my eyes. Months later I discovered that the woman hadn't even met her own goal of making it to Christmas. I cried then and still do every time I remember her smile and that look in her sad eyes.

Chapter 13

I felt I was on the mend again and as the summer started we were treated to a long string of gorgeous days. We planned a holiday in Italy, staying on the Amalfi coast. We wanted to be based first in Sorrento – so we could visit Pompeii and Herculaneum, having not been there since Grace and I first met as students – before moving to the other side of the peninsular.

It was also wonderful being back at work again, and I picked up where I had left off with regular clients much sooner than I or anyone else could have believed. Every day I worked on something. I was active. The work was complex, challenging and yet satisfying. It had a clear beginning and a pleasing end. Working was an act of defiance and there was so much to be done. Under pressure, I was getting better. I had found my rhythm and style again. The trips to India were proof of my recovery.

I saw my friends and family. These days, they came round to check that I still existed. They came to salute my recovery and help stab cancer in the back. We were all reassured. I was the man again, whole and alive. We welcomed them all to our house and it felt good to be regaining my life. The free-floating humour and wit came back to me in flashes and the words and laughter were impetuous and sudden. Conversations were joyful and purposeful, but nevertheless they were without insight and so at times I felt the tension and the dark days that were still just over my shoulder. I could sense them and sometimes they would return so I could taste the bitter blackness that still hung over me.

I could not imagine being without my family and friends. I was thinking of a future again, entertaining the possibility that this illness was finished. I started to enjoy food and drink as before: chocolate, good coffee and decent wine. I was pro-life and the living of it in the way I once did and now could again. This is what it meant to be a grown-up human being, doing what I had done for most of my life before the illness, making decisions, reforming habits. That's what grown-ups do.

Grace pored over the internet, seeking out dangerous things, bad things, things I shouldn't do, eat or drink, things that I hadn't cared about until now. We reconsidered our choices, my choices. My oncologist Dr J was our most clued-up adviser and she was always careful with her guidance. The NHS recommended a balanced diet, as did Grace. Eat well but take all things in moderation. OK, that was clear enough. So we ate well and I drank less alcohol. I embraced moderation and less generous portions. I took vitamins and other supplements along with the other drugs I still needed, such as the loperamide I required to manage the alien stoma which was forever part of me now. At times I feared the drugs would eventually capsize me and I would sink through the treacle that still flowed around my ankles.

So we were looking forward to our much-needed summer holiday in Italy. The break would serve many functions. For Grace it was a chance to get away from the last nine months of hell. For me it was my constitutional as I weaned myself off chemotherapy drugs. I was well enough and we needed to move out of our little bubble of air and into another atmosphere. Gentle walks in the sun that would warm my tired muscles; excellent Italian dining; amazing views of the Amalfi coastline and countryside; and the thrill of Roman Pompeii again.

It was wonderful to return to that magical part of the world. Together, we explored. The blue sky and the wine-dark Mediterranean invigorated our senses and nurtured our love for each other. Outdoor dinners at restaurants overlooking sea bays, hummus, fresh olives and breadsticks, pasta and seafood with a bottle of Prosecco. Nights were sweet and the streets of Sorrento busy and inviting, with wonderful smells of alfresco dining, burnt sugar and nougat. There was time to read and talk. It was delightful to be together, just in each other's company, drifting through each day.

One late afternoon, as the sun sank low in the reddening sky, we sat and watched through slit eyes as several teenagers played football on the beach under the cliff before taking turns to swim. Because of my stoma, I hadn't been swimming since my operation. Now I longed to join them in the warm water. Its surface sparkled red and orange. The beach was aglitter with pink pearls. A young girl drew a heart in the sand with a stick and a big wet woman staggered from the sea with her big wet dog.

The beach was emptying as I looked at Grace. She was golden as she slowly teased her toes in the warm, black larva sand.

We said nothing. I took photographs of the teenagers diving into the shallow water to catch balls kicked into the waves for them by their mates. Darkening silhouettes as the sun went down, laughing and gesticulating in true Napolitano style. How I envied them their athleticism. And yet I was grateful just to be there.

During those days I was always looking for a place on which to rest my eyes, to find peace and beauty and images that would not hurt me but would help remove the past few months of fear and rid me of the dark place just over my shoulder.

In Italy I often found myself shutting my eyes, feeling the sun, sensing the moment but not wanting to see again unless I found it wasn't real and I was back. I wanted to open my eyes to find myself whole again, but the hard evidence of the imprinted past wouldn't let me. Still, I was alive and I was recovering and Grace and I were together. It was like falling in love all over again, being in that place and having a future with my wife by my side.

In Ravello, walking up through the steep, tight streets, curving upwards past the old hotels with glorious rear-terraced gardens that opened up onto spectacular, sparkling sea views as the land fell away, past a runnel of grass where the early evening katydids sang, we sat on a bench to admire the beauty of the architecture. Grace slipped her hand into mine and whispered that she loved me and everything was going to be OK.

We are all creatures of habit and context. At that time I could only see what was directly in front of me. I only *wanted* to see what was directly in front of me and think of what I wanted to believe. The sky only appears blue. Beyond it we know it edges from blue to black, from black to a darker black and to a darker place, away from the atmosphere of our earth, away from the air that we need to breathe to live our lives. I thought that there was a limit to our pain. I thought that it was finite. I was sure now that it would end.

Chapter 14

My next visit to my oncologist Dr J was on 1 October, the day before our wedding anniversary. They had subjected me to a re-staging CT scan two weeks before and taken blood samples, so by the time of the appointment I was awaiting the results.

We were sitting in the Stoke Mandeville cancer clinic, close to Dr J's office. She was late for our meeting as she so often was. She tended to spend longer with her patients than she really had time for. We would take up more than our allocated time because we patients had questions and she always obliged us with a careful response. Of course she did.

This time, unusually, there were three nurses standing around outside her office. One was thumbing through some papers in a thick file; probably mine, I thought. The other two were whispering to each other and the one with her back to me turned slowly and smiled. A strange sort of half smile; sadness in her eyes that confused me. Grace read a magazine as I twisted my fingers together.

These days I never looked forward to my visits to Dr J, not because I didn't want to see her – on the contrary, she was always easy and empathetic, kind and generous with her time and careful with her answers – but because I was always frightened that her news might not be good news, might be negative or a problem for me. She always spoke quickly, as if she was late. Grace and I both suspected that she was just much smarter than we were. We found ourselves trying to keep pace with what she said. She always smiled when she greeted us and asked how I was.

Suddenly her door swung open. The nurses turned to face us as my name was called. I jumped up and walked with purpose to her office, Grace behind catching up. She always said I never waited for her. She was right, I was always eager to get into the consultation.

As before, Dr J was smiling but she immediately asked me to sit as she had some disappointing news. I went cold and as I felt the blood drain from my head. Her voice got fainter; I knew she was going to tell me something bad.

What I didn't know was just how bad.

The CT scan revealed new liver metastases. The cancer hadn't gone away; it had spread. It was in my liver.

We sat silently, crushed.

My mind was numb. I still had cancer. The cancer was now in my liver. That meant no hope. The cancer would take my life. Although I was present in that room I wasn't with anyone. I couldn't think of what it meant. It was quiet in my head. No one disturbed me. I wanted to hide, to run away again. Then the darkness rose up again and sat on my shoulder and I remember feeling how cold it was, just sitting there in that office.

I could smell my own fear on my skin. Was Grace afraid, I wondered? I didn't know except that I was the chosen one out of all those people that surrounded me. I was the one in my solo dream that ended with this new information. No one else could penetrate my dream. It was the start of something that could be bad now and worse later. Something terrifyingly new and strange had happened. I was the victim again. I didn't yet know what it meant but the ground that I had been standing on was gone from under me.

Giving me this news was the whole reason for the meeting so once it had been delivered there was little else for me to do.

Dr J had been speaking. Grace, now ashen, took copious notes. I heard words like *hope*, and possibly *more surgery*. Dr J was to meet with the team to *discuss*; it was *not necessarily as bad as we think*.

We rose all together and for a moment we looked at each other; I looked at Grace and I looked at Dr J. Perhaps we could dance – take your partners please for the... Instead we sort of shook hands and murmured our thank yous and goodbyes.

What had just happened? I couldn't remember. We left the room and turned down a corridor with our entourage. We walked side by side, muted and trembling with common danger. We were shown into a quiet room, away from everyone else, where we could sit in big, comfy armchairs. The door closed and I was alone with Grace. Her lower lip trembled and her beautiful blue eyes filled with fluid as the tears streamed down her face. She sobbed uncontrollably.

My head felt better when it was supported in my hands. I hid my face. The stream of tears poured down easily in a vertical screen as the darkness, like a cowl, rose over my shoulders to cover my bowed body.

Chapter 15

I felt fine during our Italian vacation and, when we got home, Dr J decided to maintain her assessment of my performance status as zero – indicating that I was doing well – despite the cancer spreading to my liver. And yet my CT scan result made the medics send me to have urgent MRI and PET scans of my liver. With the results of these scans, Dr J and the liver surgeons at the Churchill Hospital were to discuss my situation at the next meeting of their liver cancer multidisciplinary team, or MDT.

Meanwhile, the meeting with Mr H, the stoma reversal surgeon, was cancelled. Sadly there was going to be no reversal, not at this point anyway.

The MRI scan took place on 8 October 2013 in the radiography department of the Churchill Hospital and a week or so later Grace and I went for our meeting with Dr J to discuss the imaging results as well as the MDT outcome. The scans showed that there was metastatic disease at four sites in the liver, but at least they were confined to the liver; no others had been detected anywhere else. As planned, my case had been discussed by the

MDT a few days before. I was assured that this team of liver cancer specialists was probably the best in the country.

Well, thank goodness for that, I remember thinking, only the best for me then!

The team recommended that I should have more chemotherapy, this time using irinotecan and fluorouracil, with biological agents if deemed applicable. The idea was to try and shrink the secondary tumours on my liver to an extent that surgery might be possible. Usually, when the liver is infected with secondary cancer, there is little chance of surviving and I knew that.

The treatment would last for two months, after which I would have a re-staging CT scan and another MRI scan to see whether there had been any reduction in the growth of the metastases. Depending on the outcome of the next round of chemo, surgery might follow.

The first cycle of the new chemotherapy started the following week, back at the Stoke Mandeville cancer clinic. I was to have a PICC line fitted. This, a peripherally-inserted central catheter, is a long, thin tube that is inserted into a large vein in your arm just above the bend in your elbow. It is then pushed up or, as the nurse explained it, is *threaded through* the vein until the tip is positioned in another large vein just above your heart. I watched on the ultrasound monitor as the catheter crossed my chest and into my heart. If they miss, it ends up going down the other side of your body somewhere. Luckily they didn't. I should explain that I was given a local anaesthetic by injection, so I didn't feel any pain while the PICC line was being inserted.

I knew the nurse who performed this procedure from my previous chemotherapy treatment sessions. She was always jolly, chatty and smiley. She pretended to be a bit of a dizzy blonde (she was blonde) and I would often hear her say that she had forgotten to do this or deal with that, but actually she was just very busy. Her gentle, happy and careful approach always made me feel relaxed and I trusted her, so when she announced, looking at the monitor, that the PICC line had gone too close to my heart and she would have to pull it out a bit, my heart started to race so much it could have pushed the damn thing out in protest. Once the PICC was in the right place, she fixed the other end, outside my arm, to a special bung that was to be attached to an IV drip for my drugs.

There was always a potential problem with these catheters. I had witnessed other patients returning to the clinic to have them removed as they had become blocked and then infected, or the area around the insertion into the arm had become infected and sore. The tube could be dislodged, which worried me. I didn't like the idea of the end of the flexible tube being sucked into my beating heart where it might stop it working. I actually needed my heart to work. Without stopping. But perhaps I was just being silly. That could never happen. As a further precaution I was x-rayed to make sure the tube was in the right place. It was, thank goodness.

The PICC line was flushed weekly in between the treatment cycles and the dressing that held it in place was changed at the same time. It was impossible for me to do it myself so a district nurse had to call in to do it for me at home.

Having this line in place meant that not only could chemotherapy drugs be passed through it but blood samples could be taken from it, so I wouldn't have to have several needles stuck into my ever-hardening veins every time I was treated. I could go home with this in me and it could be left in for weeks or months. I was so happy!

The PICC line stayed in me for several weeks. I had to wear an elasticated bandage over the tube's point of entry to hold both the line and the dressing in place. It would occasionally get stained with blood and, when the site got infected, with gunk. It hurt sometimes as it was always tight, always restrictive and of course needed to be kept dry whenever I had a shower or bath. I wore a special plastic sleeve over the bandage to stop it getting wet, thus encouraging infection. But even when this was tightened at both ends, it was never really watertight.

Picture the scene: I am trying to wash my hair and the rest of myself with one hand whilst keeping the other arm elevated somewhere above my head. Grace burst into laughter when she first saw me sitting in the bath with a plastic-sleeved arm raised high above my head like a primary schoolchild trying to attract the teacher's attention to help them tie a shoe lace.

Much later, I needed to have a second PICC line put in, this time by a sister who I suspected hadn't performed the procedure many times before, despite the fact that she told me she had done "hundreds of these in her time". Her time *as what* I wasn't sure.

The procedure started well enough except that she was accompanied by an auxiliary nurse, who was lovely. Strangely, the auxiliary and I struck up a conversation about liquorice as it transpired that we both adored the rock-hard sticks of the black stuff when we were kids. As we conducted this rather absurd conversation, the sister prepared my left arm. Antiseptic applied, local anaesthetic administered, vein allocated and needle presented. She prodded and inserted the needle, withdrew the needle and tried again. And again. Her now flushed face and dark, piercing eyes hinted that she might be having a problem. Without even flinching, she decided that it was my arm that was the problem and immediately switched to the other one. She rushed round to my right side, told the auxiliary nurse to hold me, placed a large sheet of plastic under my right side and without any local anaesthetic this time, drove the needle into a vein, The auxiliary nurse was desperate to keep my attention focused on her but her open mouth and wide-eyed expression told me that perhaps this wasn't best practice. As the pain increased and blood ran down my arm and dripped noisily onto the plastic sheet on the floor, I asked if the use of an ultrasound monitor might help her guide the now inserted flexible line to its correct position. A blood-stained, blue-rubber-gloved hand swept back a wisp of black hair from sister's rather damp and flushed brow and those dark, piercing eyes closed a little more.

"Only recently-trained nurses use ultrasound," she hissed.

I lay very still and talked to the auxiliary nurse about Pontefract cakes. Had I known exactly how painful the insertion was going to be I think I would have chosen to take that one-way trip to Switzerland instead.

After my first cycle of the new drugs, Grace and I saw Dr J again on 5 November, Guy Fawkes Night. I had tolerated the irinotecan and fluorouracil chemotherapy better than I had expected and my performance status was rated at zero again. I had suffered constipation for a few days, caused by the ondansetron that I had been prescribed to combat the drugs, but things had settled down after that. However, I was feeling far more nausea; I lost my appetite and was also suffering from indigestion. Worse was the fact that my peripheral neuropathy, the pain and numbness caused by the oxaliplatin, was more troublesome and had spread to my feet and especially my toes. These hurt all the time now and prevented me from sleeping well. I moved to another room to stop waking Grace as I thrashed around at night trying to rid myself of the pain. I was prescribed yet more drugs, this time a low dose of amitriptyline to tackle the neuropathy and help me get some rest. I also needed a proton pump inhibitor to help reduce stomach acid.

I was to have the second and third cycles of treatment before being seen again by Dr J and also a repeat CT scan and liver MRI scan at the Churchill after the fourth cycle. The liver team would then review the effects of the treatment and, if there was no response, then definitive liver resection, in other words surgery, would be considered.

I was fitted with a pump as all these drugs needed to be slowly dripped into me over two days. It wasn't really a pump in engineering terms, but a cylinder about the size of a drink can with a tube stuck in it and attached to my PICC line. Its bulk meant that, to carry it, it hung from a cradle strapped round my waist. It would be like this for the duration of the treatment. The drugs were placed in a balloon inside the transparent cylinder and as they emptied into me, the balloon deflated. When the balloon was empty, I had to go back to the clinic to have it removed, my PICC line flushed with saline, my PICC entry point checked and the dressing changed. None of this was painful but having the contraption attached to me meant we couldn't really go out, and we had to return to the hospital every week during this period until I had the pump removed.

Chapter 16

Since that day, the day I was told about the secondary cancer in my liver, I had begun to consider that my future was possibly not very bright.

I could not imagine not being alive and yet that's what I was now beginning to think. My mind constantly moved into that dark place. What would it be like for my family when I wasn't there? I couldn't formulate an idea of the future. My thoughts ran ahead of my reality all the time. I felt the images of my future, our future, slip away every time I tried to conjure them up. My mouth would dry just as the tears started to well. I had no grip on myself, let alone on my future. I was no longer in control.

I rehearsed the possibilities but I didn't like them. They were cruel and hurtful and I felt like a beaten dog. They gnawed at me, worried me and scared me. I told myself that it wasn't happening to me. It wasn't true. It was a nightmare that I would wake from and the dark place would disappear.

There were other times when I refused to bend to those thoughts, when I was determined to see a viable future. I could face up to the challenge and I would beat this and win. The path I had to follow was obvious. Endure the treatment, face the surgery, accept the love, be positive and all would be well.

I had been sceptical but now I had no choice as everything had already been configured. My oncologist Dr J knew. She was clued up. She had knowledge and she would do what was right, what was for the best. She would tell me the truth, the possibilities if positive as well at the probabilities if they were negative. She was our informant and she was a careful and honest woman.

At times I couldn't cope with any of it. I would catch myself in the mirror, my eyes red from crying, my skin blotchy and my hair thin and lacklustre. My image was there in the mirror but it wasn't really me – was it? I often felt nauseous and tired and my feet hurt but I couldn't say much; no one wanted to hear the story of pain and misery again, not again.

"How are you today?"

Fine, thank you.

"You look – so well."

Thank you.

I had shrivelled to half my size. I became a gnawed-at, crumbling, crying child. My game was up. What did I need to do to end it? My head hurt, I wanted to die and I felt like I needed to vomit from it but I couldn't. This is what I often thought but by mistake it would come out of my mouth differently as speech: *I am not going to die.*

I needed someone to scream at or something to smash or dirt to dig or just to sleep and sleep and sleep. I couldn't talk to anyone about this, so I told Grace. The air would crackle and fizz and my brain boiled and writhed as I tried to explain what I felt. White flashes of hysterical fear and pain made my head throb.

I would try to formulate my thoughts, compose a response to her questions. I tried to arrive at an intellectual position about death, if that was what was going to happen, to grieve then in advance, in preparation. I didn't know how to cope and yet people would say how well I was coping. What did they know that I didn't? What did they see that I obviously couldn't see? It was all opaque to me.

At a dinner someone held my arm and whispered, "You are doing so well, coping with this." I felt my legs give way as my magic drained from me, my power dissolved like salt in tepid water. I felt weak and vulnerable yet again. I wanted to sit in the corner and be hugged back to strength, put by our log fire and warmed back to life as it used to be.

I was becoming different. The children had noticed it and commented on it to Grace. *Dad's not as much fun as he used to be.* The fun had been sucked out of me. What did they expect? Even Woody Allen was funnier – hell's teeth, I really had lost it! I was different and I was very conscious of it. How could I have avoided it? I saw the future as a huge, inert mountain that I was trying to climb, but the mountain got bigger every day I tried to climb it. The summit was somewhere out of view, masked by thick, dark clouds. Was that where I was heading? Those clouds were at times like slabs of cold slate, grey-black shards, where the rain and wind swirled, hysterical and angry. Sometimes at night, in the sky above the clouds, the moon would slowly disappear behind the grey slate and I would be cast into darkness, alone and cold. Was that where I was truly heading?

Sometimes, I would find myself lying down quietly on a sofa somewhere in the house with my eyes closed, a little estranged from myself, thinking of our apartment by the sea. I loved the sea. I loved being by it and in it. Would there be a time when I would never see it again? Never swim in it again? Feel the salty spray from it on a windy day again? It was a chance for my imagination to revisit my past, reconsider what I had done to deserve my plight, what I might have done to avoid the situation I now found myself in.

I overturned each stone in my head, inspected every nook and cranny of my life before drifting back to the sea that I loved, only to find myself wading further into the waves, feeling them suddenly crash over me, over my head, under the water, face down as the water pulled me down until the light faded and the sea suddenly became calm; and so did I.

There were other times when I would find myself in a garden, a blank garden with blank trees. No leaves. Our friends from Miami called them naked trees. They used to visit us in very early springtime when there were no leaves and always loved the bleak nudity of the trees in England – something they never experienced in Florida, of course. How I wished at that moment that I could escape there, be flown on a magic Turkish carpet to the heart of Miami for the sun and green trees and peace and freedom. But the trees in our garden were skeletal; some were bleached sepia and white or charred black – all having been struck by a cancerous lightning bolt – yet they were all still standing erect, swaying in their death agony.

I would lie, stretched out on the grass under those trees and look up though their branches, up their lengths to the point where the tip touched those slabs of cold, slate sky. What were they pointing at, I wondered? Where was I supposed to look and for what? I lay there for a long time as the tips of the trees swayed and the slabs of grey passed by.

I was not spared the violence of knowledge about what might happen. I could no longer speak nor laugh. Tears were easy and sadness bountiful but I still could not see beyond the tips of those trees. I wanted to learn how to articulate my thoughts about my future. I was at the beginning of what could well be a new end to my life and the impact on me was beginning to have a grave mental as well as physical effect. There was no sun that fell on me as I lay in our garden. I was in the midst of derangement. I would ask myself out loud: What is happening to me? What has happened to me? What might still happen to me?

I mouthed the words as I gazed up through those branches. *I am in trouble, I have some bad news. The cancer has spread to my liver and people don't survive secondary cancer in their liver. It is not yet known whether I will survive or not. I need to have part of my liver taken away and then we shall see. I will undergo an operation. I may or may not live. I don't know yet what it means in terms of my future. Do I have one or not? What problems might there be? What will the side effects be? It's a very uncertain time for me and my family. This is a shock but I am strong, I think.*

And I look so well. Everybody tells me I look so well, but they don't understand. They don't know what is going on inside my body and they don't know what is going on in my brain. I may need some help after the operation – assuming I survive the operation – but I don't know what sort of help I may need. We will have to see. I will let you know.

I will let you know.

I will.

Another time, I found myself floating in a bed of soft pillows, high above those trees. It was quiet but I didn't know why. However, the silence quietened the demon on my shoulder and reduced the darkness there until it was only misty grey. I was stuck in those pillows and yet they supported my anxiety. Was I already dead? Was I hallucinating? I had to feel the pillows to make sure that I was still alive. They were soft, like clouds might be. I looked over the sides, down between the trees and saw someone lying on the grass, gazing up at me. I waved. They didn't. Why don't they wave? I sometimes slept for a few minutes at a time to wake up and remember that this wasn't a dream. It was real and I was in the real world. The dark place would descend and surround me as the demon crept back up onto my shoulder.

Chapter 17

Going out anywhere was now a risk. Travelling was a hazard. As the treatment continued and I went through the next two cycles, I was more aware of the possibilities of infection and the potential outcome if I became neutropenic. Most nights were sleepless. Sometimes I felt strangely exhilarated and super-charged. Maybe I could live without any sleep; maybe I could live forever with a pump permanently fixed to my waist as well as my stoma and a plastic pipe looped round my body into my heart. I could put everything I needed to live in that pump. Half a bottle of gin before bed, a milk shake for breakfast, a liquid protein supplement for lunch. If I got the amounts right and used up the calories generated, I wouldn't even need my bloody stoma.

I was kidding myself of course, but the PICC line did have its uses. If I became neutropenic it would allow me to have a direct blood transfusion. Other patients had easily been given platelets and antibiotics through them.

Emily, our eldest daughter, was working on her doctorate in clinical psychology at Stoke Mandeville Hospital with both the spinal unit teams – renown across the world for their rehabilitation work – as well as in their cancer clinic. I was having my usual treatment at the cancer clinic in the late morning. Around lunch time, volunteers came round to take our sandwich order. There was a choice as long as you liked cheese or tuna in white bread, and a fruit yogurt. I always struggled to find the fruit in mine.

I knew Emily was working at the main hospital that day and she texted me to ask if we could have lunch together. She found me in one of the open bays mid-treatment, which meant I was snuggled up in my large reclining plastic armchair, newspaper open at the crossword on one side and my Kindle on the other with my sandwich in one hand and a carton of orange juice perched on a little side table.

Emily pulled up a chair and unwrapped her lunch, and we ate and chatted together. The nurses started to gather at the reception desk and were looking at me quite quizzically, whispering to each other and on occasion walking over to ask if I was alright, to which I replied that I was and thanked them. When we had finished lunch, Emily packed up her things and left, saying goodbye to any staff who were around. No sooner had she gone than two of them raced over and sat with me, one held my hand and both looked very concerned.

"Are you alright?" one asked with a deep frown.

"Yes, thank you," I replied, a little bemused. They weren't usually that concerned about a patient unless he was howling in pain.

"Are you coping with the treatment? We know how traumatic the latest news must have been."

I didn't understand their concern and asked them what they meant.

"Well, to have one of the clinical psychologists come and see you surprised us, as you seemed to be coping with things very well. So we were quite worried."

They didn't know that Emily was my daughter. It hadn't occurred to them, despite the same surname, and they hadn't even suspected when she gave me a parting kiss on the cheek. I wasn't sure who was more relieved, them or me.

Grace's birthday was just after the last meeting with Dr J, back in November. It was a subdued time for me, yet we decided to go out for the day. The effort was so worth it, the rewards obvious. Pleasures had to be won and, when they were, we were both the better for it.

We had lunch, tick. We went for a walk, tick. We had afternoon tea, tick. I drove and we savoured the normality of it all throughout the whole day, like dark chocolate truffle melting slowly in our mouths. As we walked in the Chiltern Hills, it was on ground carpeted with autumn leaves over a chalky underlay. The views were vast and wide, even though the low clouds and distant rain reduced the clarity of the panorama. For thousands of years, people had come here to see this same view. They must have marvelled at it and loved it and felt healthy, happy and fulfilled, just as we did.

For that moment anyway.

The walk was good, tick.

We felt so far away from all our troubles, protected by this complicated and bizarre zone we were in at that time. We watched the grey smudge in the sky as the rain clouds edged closer. Most of the time these days I hardly knew where I was or what I was doing. I had been in a dream-like state and going forward into the future seemed just as dream-like. Now we stood there in the Chilterns and watched the rain arrive. We could have been waiting for a bomb to go off. It would have been a perfect place to watch a mushroom cloud rise majestically into the rain-streaked sky and blow us into oblivion.

Our lunch was a feast of salad and cheeses, Parma ham and olives, fresh bread and rich butter. We walked back along the grassy path. The rain had abated and so we sat for a while on a bench dedicated to somebody's recently-lost but still-loved father. The bench had been placed awkwardly in front of a thatched cottage, now apparently abandoned. There were no survivors there. I remember we huddled together, as close as possible, to make ourselves so small that the cold couldn't get us, nor the demons that sat more boldly on my shoulders. Our coats wrapped tightly round us, our scarves and gloves sealed off the windy chill. No one else was around. We were there for us, at the heart of that terrible game that needed to be played out, whatever the outcome. The game had to be played until the final whistle was blown and the score known. We weren't spectators. The spectators were not on our hill, they were far away but they were there watching and waiting to see the outcome of our game as well.

The tea house was at the bottom of the hill through the woods. The tea was welcomingly hot and the window seat warm. We drained our tea pot. We had a lovely day. Together.

My main client asked me if I could do some more work, a follow-up assessment. The request came as a relief and the work kept me busy during late November and into the lead-up to Christmas.

We decided to have a proper family portrait taken and arranged a photographic session for all five of us, using the lounge as our backdrop. Its white shutters, New-Hampshire-style, and deep-seated cream sofas seemed to make it the perfect location. My niece's husband is a good photographer and he offered to manage the modelling session. It was a lovely excuse for the girls to be at home with us, and to dress up together in black and creams. I wore a pink, thin-striped shirt. It matched my blotchy dry skin, florid face and sore eyes. Alex, the photographer, lit the various scenes expertly enough to mask the condition of my face. Black-and-white photographs seemed so much gentler than colour. It was a lovely time and we all treasured the moment. I needed to have photographs of us all together. It was important for my peace of mind.

The weather was getting colder as the autumn slipped into winter. I started wearing thermal vests, wrapping up in scarves and even wearing a hat; I never used to wear one before. It was important that I didn't catch any colds or flu while I was being given the next five cycles of chemotherapy. I measured my temperature daily and also every time I felt slightly under the weather. The effects of the treatment and my physical and mental state were beginning to affect my health. My temperature sometimes tripped over the killer number 38C, but normally slid back down within an hour or so. A temperature over 37C would lead to a phone call and immediate hospitalisation, but so far we were OK, we were saved. The scares I got from even slight temperature fluctuations gave me a sick feeling in my stomach, an introduction to the sudden fear of a potential major melt down. We knew the danger. We knew it would be serious and we knew it *would probably occur* sometime and possibly soon.

As the month progressed many people around us seemed to be coughing and complaining of the cold and their aches and pains. My second cycle of chemo started at the clinic according to plan on 18 November. I needed more saline than usual, new bungs for my PICC and a change of dressing. Was the site getting infected? My arm ached more than usual and a red sore patch had developed.

The dark evenings were depressing, but at least the log burner kept me warm as it rained cold wet sheets outside. My neuropathy was more painful in the cold. My finger-tips still hurt a little and even with nice thick woolly socks, my toes ached. We moved around the house, strange characters in a strange play, crammed together in the warm places. Bed was best. Despite the unreality of it all, Grace continued as ever with her love and acts of generosity and kindness.

December arrived. My third cycle of chemotherapy began on the 2nd and the pump, now empty, was removed on the 4th. I had time in between those relentless cycles of chemo treatment (avoiding going anywhere, avoiding the cold, avoiding the garden, avoiding people) to paint more. I told myself quite often that *I was an artist.* Of sorts. I dabbled with paint very much as an amateur, but I had exhibited my work multiple times and had sold a few pictures. My objective was to build up a decent portfolio of watercolours and oils and then create my own website to tout my wares online.

My studio was one of our five bedrooms. It didn't have a bathroom attached like the others. It was north-facing and so was perfect for painting in oils, but it was also large enough to take a comfortable leather sofa and a rather large TV, which I had managed to con Grace into letting me buy. She said it looked much smaller in the shop than it did when it was installed in what then developed into my very own *man cave*.

Opening the door to my studio was like walking into another world, a world in which I could create imaginary vistas, scenarios and people. The season didn't matter when I was in there. It could have been any day, anywhere, any hour of any day, light or night. I would sit and think and draw and paint and plan and make art and assess my work. In that room was a history of my journeys and thoughts and wishes. Everything that I had set in motion through brush and colour was there. It was a complex mixture of pleasures. When I breathed in, the warmth and smell of paint would unpack around me. I felt deep affection for that room during those days. It was me and my escape. Sometimes, however, I was afraid of it. Would it always be there even if I wasn't? I could lose it and it would no longer be part of me if I wasn't there. At those times and in that room I yearned for my life to be as it had been before.

I usually worked in silence. When I did put on a CD I usually chose classical opera or depressing ballads. Grace couldn't bear to listen to anything sad, but she didn't tell me that at the time. How I must have made her suffer! The space in my studio wasn't large but it was mine and it was warm against those wintery days. The light was a photographer's light, pale whitish grey and perfectly even, as long as you sat by the window. I liked being there but others would come and stand by the door, almost not daring to enter the space, the artist's inner sanctum. With the door closed you would not know it existed. You could walk past it quite easily, but I often kept the door open with the latest picture facing the landing so that, on passing, I could see it, scrutinise it and remind myself of the need to complete it, or change something in it or try to repair any poor brush strokes.

My visual world of painting and drawing, real or otherwise, had not lost its edge but instead was rekindled with vigour, determination and hope. It became perpetual and cognitive. Indeed, my compass shifted and my eyes became more focused on the need to create new and more pictures. My work would progress with speed at times too. I would not let what skill I had become redundant. If I lost my ambition to paint, I was fearful that I would lose my focus on life and therefore my hope. I therefore stayed busy, never letting my easel be without its companion canvas. In bursts, I was frenetically active. Ideas got painted and projects developed, but I decided I wasn't going to exhibit again. I was going to go private. In one brush stroke I decided I was going to paint *my* way, for me alone. I was going to paint to ensure that I kept myself alive so that our family could continue. Our family unit of five was like a solid, geometric mass of coloured, three-dimensional paint. We had texture and dimension, weight and surface, patina and form. That was all that mattered to me and I grasped it with both hands.

My ambition was concrete and different from any other ambition I had ever felt the need to achieve. I needed my family to help me secure that ambition though. I knew I couldn't make it happen by myself. I wasn't in control but I could, with all the people who loved me, who were looking out for me, who were treating me, possibly get through all this and reach my goal. I couldn't change the terms of my condition through my own will, but what I could do was change my approach. Painting in my man cave during that cold December helped me realise that.

My blood tests showed I was just about OK so the fourth chemotherapy cycle began according to plan. I had the usual preparation and retained my pump until it was removed on 18 December, just before my next CT and MRI scans. The build-up to the scans was always stressful and I became irritable, sharp and bad tempered. The closer the day came, the worse I got. Grace took most of this without complaint. I knew it was hurting her and yet I seemed incapable of doing anything about it. Of course it wasn't the scans that I dreaded, but the results, which were to be delivered by Dr J two weeks later, after Christmas.

I remember Christmas as a bit of a blur. I felt exhausted and we weren't really inclined to celebrate. The appointment with Dr J the week after Christmas hung so heavily over my bowed head that it hurt. Every time I lifted it, my brain struck the dreaded date and I heard it clang against my cranium, ringing noisily as my forehead throbbed. We seemed to barely function through the whole of that festive season. Our friends were stoical and we saw many of them, but the mood was sullen and their ashen faces no doubt matched mine.

My cancer seemed to move so fast it scarcely allowed us time to look at it, let alone get used to it. I hadn't seen it as a high-speed disease. I didn't perceive it as possibly ending in a mass motorway pile up, but it certainly wasn't allowing us to travel in the slow lane and watch the scenery glide serenely past us or admire the view.

I often thought that I could be in big trouble, and if I was, then what was going to happen? Sometimes it seemed more frightening than others. Was I going to manage this or not? Was I going to survive this or not and, if not, then what? Was this next scan going to be manageable and benign? Later, would we be able to look back at all this and laugh? Over that Christmas we managed to maintain the thin façade of a functioning family during what for most was a joyous time. We acted as others did and as we used to do in the past, but to plan ahead, go away or go on holiday seemed wrong and beyond us. Should we have just abandoned the pretence? It might have been easier to stop and not try to live a normal life anymore.

At times I got stressed and angry and my outbursts and tears would upset Grace and the family, if they were around. I was frightened and yet I didn't know why. I had not had any bad news. I had not had the results, good or bad. They could be fine. I had not been so frightened before, so why was it happening now? I tried to brush off the dark demon that I often found sitting on my shoulder during that Christmas. Grace was my balance, my steady supporting rock that I leant on whenever the darkness descended but she couldn't keep that up forever. *I am here for you. We all love you. We are safe at home.* She would repeat these phrases like a mantra. I knew she was right, but I found her reassurance difficult to accept. I used to sit on the sofa next to her and we would look at each other and she would inspect my face, searching for the rays of hope that she wanted desperately to see in me. Yet all I could do was respond with silence or tears and quite often both as I sobbed into her protective arms.

When I got angry my voice would get louder than usual. I sometimes couldn't control the volume. I blamed the demon on my left shoulder for that. I would broadcast my anger that was really my frustration that was actually my fear. I would complain about minor things, from food to the *BBC News*, from my inability to complete the newspaper crossword to the temperature of my mug of tea. We would have a quiet little low-temperature argument perhaps. I would make an excuse to leave the room – to empty my stoma bag, perhaps – so I could shake off the anger and move out of the dark place. My mood at times felt vicious inside of me as I tried to talk to the demon on my left shoulder. The choice was always between roaring at him so loud in the back of my throat that it ripped off the skin, or complete, full-on hysterics.

Eventually, I would regain my composure and return. Grace would always know what I had been thinking. It was killing me, I thought, one way or another. It *was* killing me.

My hair might have thinned out somewhat, but I thought I looked quite well for a man full of toxins. You wouldn't have thought I was ill, would you? I would gaze into Grace's very beautiful blue eyes. When we first met, it was her eyes that had been the main draw.

My weight was back to where it was before the surgery. My skin had become more translucent and in places sore and red, but perhaps it wasn't too bad for a man who was being slowly poisoned by medics. Darker crescents developed under my eyes. Sleep deprivation. I was often woken with the uncomfortable knowledge that I had a pump attached to me. I had to keep it wedged under my pillow so that a sudden movement didn't wrench the PICC from my arm.

We existed during that Christmas, trying to enjoy the festivities, willing ourselves to do the normal things as we always had done. We were heads-down and busy with all the chores that queued up to be done. We decorated the tree, cooked the turkey, dressed up for a gathering. I talked to the clinical psychologist who we had on tap in the shape of our daughter Emily. It was good therapy, but it wasn't our best Christmas.

We went to our appointment at the Stoke Mandeville cancer clinic following the scans. Grace and I were due to see Dr J for the results and then I was to have my next cycle of drugs. The day before, the usual blood samples had been taken, so we were waiting for those results as well. I remember parking outside the clinic. We sat in the car. I couldn't move. I rested my head in my hands. A Radio 4 programme was on somewhere in the car and the weak winter sun filtered through the windscreen. The skin on my hands felt sore and looked it. I felt tired and suddenly panicky.

Another patient drew up alongside us. Parking was always difficult in that place unless you were lucky. A woman got out of the car and went to open the passenger door. A man struggled to get out. Pale yellow skin. Late sixties perhaps. He looked unsteady and not particularly well. We grew used to seeing older, sicker-looking patients amble slowly and with difficulty into the clinic. They didn't see us and yet we saw all of them every time. I sighed and a feeling of nausea swept over me. I looked at Grace and she smiled at me, a thin, sad sort of smile. We both knew that we had to go through with the appointment. There was never any choice, but I always dreaded the outcomes. I could feel the darkness descend over my shoulder as we each opened our car doors and edged out into the chilly morning.

We entered the clinic and joined the queue to check in. I was alert to every awful nuance around me. I made a wish, but when I turned to look over my shoulder the demon was still sitting there. Why couldn't I be wrapped up in multiple layers of cling film, totally protected from all that was happening? I wanted some armour and for it to be impenetrable. Where was my fairy godmother now when I needed her? I had made my wish but she seemed to have bloody well gone on holiday somewhere, in the warm sun no doubt, far away in Fairyland. I was in the queue, edging towards the receptionist. I could have turned around and left, not checked in. Would anyone have known or cared?

Morning. Name please. Have you got your letter and who is your appointment with?

Chapter 18

stared at the CT scan results that Dr J handed me. The scan specification was "chest-abdomen-pelvis with contrast". Dr J was talking somewhere in the distance at high speed as she always did. I caught a glimpse of Grace's fingers, her pen and note pad. She was writing furiously as she always did. I was trying to concentrate as my heart raced, as it always did.

Comparison study:

1. *There has been an interval increase in the size of the liver metastases; most obviously the peripheral lesion in segment VII now measures 15mm compared to 8mm previously.*

2. *No lung metastases.*

3. *No lymphadenopathy.*

4. *Unremarkable spleen, pancreas, adrenals and kidney.*

5. *No bone metastases.*

Conclusion: internal progression in liver metastases; segments II-III appear to be free of the disease.

We delved a little deeper into what all this meant, though it was pretty obvious. Anatomists divide the liver into lobes and further into eight functional segments, numbered I to VIII. A metastasis on my segment VI had actually reduced from 24 to 18mm. Good; the chemotherapy must have worked. A segment VII lesion was essentially unchanged at 28mm but the peripheral segment VII lesion, as mentioned in the report, had enlarged slightly from 18 to 23mm. Er, hang on! That wasn't what the comparison study said. The report said it had grown, yes, but from 8 to 15mm. Now I was being told that it had actually expanded from 18 to 23mm? Confusion had already clouded my brain and I could tell it was clouding other brains in the room too. Still the conversation continued. The segment VIII lesion was unchanged at 44mm.

The most important outcome of all this was what I wanted to know. Dr J as always provided us with the clarity we sought. First, in effect there had been only minimal change in the size of the different cancerous metastases; and second, there were still none in the left lobe, which was made up of segments II and III.

I didn't know it at the time, but those last few words, *still none in the left lobe*, were the ones that were to save my life.

The blood tests showed that my critical cell counts were down. For this reason, chemotherapy would cease. There wasn't much point continuing with it anyway, as it hadn't really worked. I went to have my PICC line removed. The area around the insertion was swollen and painful so I needed to have some major attention anyway. The last thing I needed was to develop a thrombosis; a blood clot forming in the vein at the tip of the line could have been fatal. It was often said *it won't be the cancer that will kill you, it'll be all the other side effects that will do it.*

The PICC line had been taped and covered with a dressing to hold it in place. One of the usual nurses who worked along the corridor from the chemotherapy bays took it out. The process was quick and painless. She said, "Brace yourself and stay still," as she gently pulled it out. I felt it re-trace its original journey up into my heart as it slid back along all the veins from my heart, across my chest and down and out of my arm. It only took a few minutes and then I was done. We said goodbye and went home.

Chapter 19

Although my chemotherapy had been cancelled I still had an appointment to see Dr J at the Stoke Mandeville clinic on New Year's Eve. That morning I woke with a fever. Grace immediately reached for the thermometer and, sure enough, my temperature had dramatically broken through the magic point and was now over 39C. After much bustling around and hasty bag packing, we drove straight to our local hospital's A&E department. Luckily, I had my NHS medical certificate with me; flashing that at reception got me around the triage process so I was spared the usual several hours of waiting to get even that far.

I was immediately segregated. It was clear that I had become neutropenic and therefore the slightest infection would be of concern. Without undressing I was bundled onto a trolley and wheeled around the corner and into an isolation room. That's what it said on the door. In hindsight it should have read, *Forgotten Prisoner Cell*. An IV drip was attached to my arm and connected to saline solution and a concoction of antibiotics. I told Grace to go home. There was no need for her to stay as I was in A&E in a top-rated hospital and would be well looked after by the highly trained and caring staff.

She left begrudgingly. It *was* New Year's Eve after all.

There I lay in the isolation room, fully dressed, with no blanket, no nurse and no water to drink. In fact, no anything except an emergency buzzer. This consisted of a button connected to a lead that disappeared somewhere under the trolley. Once the antibiotics had run out, I pressed the button and waited, expecting a flurry of activity from concerned staff who, I supposed, would either attach more drugs or saline drips or perhaps remove the lot and let me get changed into hospital garb.

No one came. I pressed the buzzer again with the same lack of result. After a few hours, I gave up pressing the silent buzzer and lay there in despair. It was dark now. I knew it was dark because as the main curtains hadn't been closed I could see the orange glow from the car park lights through the net curtains. Without a blanket I was beginning to feel cold. I couldn't move because of the catheter in my arm and the empty antibiotic bag above me, so I could neither reach my mobile phone nor get to the door to call a nurse. Also, I couldn't go for a pee.

I tried to sleep, but now the wind had got up and the old, aluminium-framed sash window had slipped open. The net curtains were being tossed about as the howling wind blew straight into the room. I had missed New Year's Eve. Now it was 1 January 2014 and I was lying on a bloody trolley with no blanket on a cold and windy night, and I was totally incapable of doing anything about it. I was so numb and tired that when Dr J strode into the room, just after nine in the morning, I thought I was in a dream.

She had been expecting me for my appointment at the clinic the day before. Grace had rung her to explain the situation and as any truly caring and professional doctor would have done, she rushed over to the hospital to find me lying in my clothes on that trolley, with no cover over me and in a freezing cold room. I was so grateful I would have hugged her had it not been for that bloody catheter. I wasn't sure if she was horrified at the total lack of care to which I had been subjected or the fact that I could have been in a much worse state than I was.

Medically, I was well enough. The antibiotics had worked and, having now been provided with a couple of blankets, I felt warmer. What now occupied my mind was the remembered image of my wonderful oncologist standing precariously on an old metal chair as she struggled desperately to close the dropped and twisted aluminium sash window of that prison cell. Although she continued to apologise for my neglect, it wasn't her fault and I repeatedly told her so. I caught her eye and gave her a look of forgiveness. We could now both at least smile and see the black humour in the situation.

I was diagnosed with neutropenic sepsis – an infection due to weakened immunity, caused by my low white blood cell count – and, after a further course of antibiotics, I was discharged four days later with a few packets of the antibiotic co-amoxiclav and some paracetamol. Yet another happy experience at the A&E department at my local hospital had been firmly committed to memory in my aching head.

It was my birthday the following Thursday, the day before I was due to meet the team of surgeons who were to carry out my liver operation, if it happened. We wanted to mark my birthday and of course we were marking something else as well. The children came round and we made a toast. It was less of a toast to celebrate a birthday than it was a wish that all would go well. *To us all and to what will come.*

We needed to make sense of what that might be. We said it out loud. Grace and I sat together and discussed the questions we would ask. We discussed what we hoped our future might look like but didn't dare to discuss the alternative scenarios. We made a list. We talked about the things we knew. We talked about the reasons we loved each other and the building blocks of our past relationship and long happy marriage. Ours was a long-time love affair, shaped to each other with our minds annexed to each other's. Grace for me was a psychic extension of myself, one that generated similar patterns of being and thinking and loving, as I was for her. It was as familiar and regular as breathing but it could all suddenly disappear, overnight, on an operating table.

It could be over in a heartbeat.

We talked about our real friends and why we loved them. Old friends as well as new ones. We talked about our children, our three golden girls, and why we adored each one of them, equally but for different reasons. It was like construction work, building on our thoughts accumulated more solidarity as it went. The possible operation was hard to speak about. We didn't know yet what was or wasn't going to be possible let alone what the outcome could be. All we knew were a few facts. The facts were:

1. If I had the operation I was going to have most of my liver removed.

2. I might die.

3. I might live a little longer.

4. *I might live a lot longer.*

It was an ugly combination of medical observations and unsupported and unverifiable predictions. Tied up in it all were statistics about similar cases before mine, and a measure of hope.

That evening I felt exhausted and collapsed on the sofa around eight o'clock. As I lay, I thought of life, my life. I thought of Grace and the girls and their lives without me. I got upset again about why this was happening to me, to us, to them. It was a dark and cold January night. It was my birthday, maybe my last birthday. I thought of things I should have been doing, finishing the list of questions for the doctors, checking the time of the appointment and seeing that I had several pound coins for the hospital's insatiable parking meter. But mostly I concentrated on staring into space through a film of moisture.

Grace told me that I should be positive, be strong; it was all going to be fine. She could see that I didn't believe her. She was telling me things that I knew weren't necessarily true. I could tell by her beautiful blue eyes and her nodding and murmuring kindnesses. I gave up protesting but it continued to upset and annoy me as she nagged away at me until I agreed. The fact that I could die seemed at that point, during that conversation, to be irrelevant. OK, so what if I was going to die? Was I in denial about the facts and Grace not?

The mental preparation for that meeting was like trying on different suits of armour. What if they said this? What if they offered an alternative? What if there wasn't any option? If it was bad news it would be almost impossible to avoid. I was no longer even conscious of who I was by the time I needed to sleep. I didn't want to go to the meeting the next day. I wanted to stay at home, stay in bed, pull the covers over me and be invisible. The dark place came over my shoulder again and I found myself holding onto Grace like you would a lamp post in the fog for fear of getting lost. I needed her to hold me. The same person that I had held so many times before when she needed me to, had to hold me then, tight, firm, warm and secure.

I would have done anything to rid myself of the dark place that night. I wanted to be a spirit, to change into something else, become a different being or shape. If I had been water I would have changed into wood, or if wood into the wind, and flown horizontally into an alternative dimension.

But none of this was possible.

The following morning at nine o'clock, we left the house and drove to the hospital.

Chapter 20

I signed the consent form. My agreement to go ahead with the liver operation was thus given at the meeting with the liver surgeons on 10 January 2014. The consultant Mr M led the team. Grace was with me as always. There were three of them with us in a small, warm room somewhere in the bowels of the hospital. One of the medics sat on the table and swung his legs mesmerisingly backwards and forwards as he locked his arms behind him and spread his hands to support his body. Another stood with his arms folded, shirt sleeves rolled up. The third and youngest of the three sat on a wooden chair at a desk where he tapped away on his laptop. Together they informed us of the pending procedure, the risks they expected and the hoped-for outcome. Grace took notes, as did the doctor with the laptop. I watched them. They looked like they were competing with each other.

This surgery was potential destruction. It could mean the obliteration of my liver – but worse, it could be the obliteration of my life. This was where we now were. There was no deserving or undeserving. No better no worse. Outside, the New Year had just begun but now I didn't know whether I would see the end of the month, let alone the end of the year. I remember thinking that it was all irrelevant, a stupid waste of time, money and effort. As the cold January air and the whole of nature outside was indifferent to me, so was I to it.

This operation was suddenly the one to fear. As I sat there in my descending fog, trying to shuffle my feet in the treacle, my mind became more confused as the shock of what I was being told blistered around my head. I was silenced by their words and could not frame a sentence with any meaning. I did try and work out what it all meant as they spoke but it got lost every time in my mental pea-souper. Slowly the dark place came again.

The medics had a plan. They had discussed my case, studied the scans and debated the results. Surgery was now presented to us as my only chance of survival. I was to get a shot at the knife. The cancer cells that had escaped from the tumour in my colon and settled in my liver hadn't responded sufficiently to the last lot of chemotherapy. They hadn't lain down and died, and so the blade was to be the way to resolution. As scientists, Grace and I wanted to know more about the procedure and yet, when I heard the first words regarding the removal of at least 60 percent of my liver, the cold sweat trickled carelessly down my neck, I stopped listening and spun out easily and quietly into vagueness.

The chief knife wielder sat swinging his legs. He doled out the facts and talked freely and eloquently about what was going to happen. We didn't find it necessary to quiz him but repeated his words like clever little parrots, agreeing and nodding appropriately, hanging on his words as if with deep understanding. We were like bewitched children, under the consultant's magic spell. My life was totally dependent on his words of Merlin-like wisdom, the precise movements of his magic wand and his supernatural powers of healing.

His words were delivered with conscious care and a clear desire not to embellish, but remain clinical and factual. We understood the importance of clear communication in such situations and our unbiased attitude towards it. There was no room for false hope, nor scope for misunderstanding. I tried not to show too much fear but instead to focus on understanding the enormity of the situation I was in. I nearly allowed this to go spectacularly awry when I asked him early on in the conversation what my chances of survival were.

The surgeons were the best in the country, a great team; Dr J had told us that. They had the best tools, steady hands and an exquisite sense of immense precision. They were craftsmen. I just hoped their craft skills hadn't been acquired in lace making or woodwork. I took a long look at the leg-swinging consultant as he eye-balled me. I wondered how risk-aware or risk-averse he was. Did he go sky-diving at the weekends without a parachute? Or was he the type to look three times before crossing a quiet road?

He had an air of relaxed confidence and I suspected (and hoped) that he had done this procedure before. The liver is not easy to operate on. It is in a rather awkward position in the abdomen, with a lot of blood vessels running in and out of it. I decided he probably knew the layout pretty well and could find where most things were. This, after all, was *his domain* and I was merely his guest at the table.

Occasionally the conversation drifted into more technical areas and I was fascinated with the way he would bring the conversation back to the basic level that he expected us to comprehend. There was a slight intake of breath, a change in the swing of his legs or a slight smile from the left side of his moving lips. I actually found him comforting and calming and, on balance, judged his expertise to outweigh my fears. He said that there was little option but to operate and if I was agreeable they would book me in at a time some weeks ahead to ensure I was in the best possible state of health.

He told me that there were several things I should be totally aware of before undergoing the surgery:

1. *I might die on the table.* Well, that's pretty standard rhetoric, but up to three percent dying during the operation seemed to me pretty bloody high statistically.

2. *If they find the cancer has spread to the other lobe or worse to other parts of the body, they might either sew me back up and tell me later that there was no point, or*

3. *They might remove other bits of me in the hope that they could save me.*

4. *(Finally, 4!) It might all go fine and the whole thing be a total success.*

I remember thinking that the last of these was my preferred outcome, so I told them that, if I was being asked to choose, I would plumb for No 4.

The liver is a rather large organ which lies on the right-hand side of the upper abdomen, just under your rib cage. It is rather important to your health. An unhealthy liver, especially one with cancer, can and probably will result in your early demise. I knew this and it scared the hell out of me. One of the things the liver does is to produce bile, which flows down a bile duct to your intestine where it mixes with food to aid digestion. Until it's needed, bile is stored in the gall bladder, which is very much part of your liver, located on the right.

The liver comes in two main parts, a small left lobe and a larger right lobe. My big positive was that only one of the lobes (though it was the large one) had been infected and this fact was to save my life. The liver receives blood from the heart through the hepatic artery and from the gut via the hepatic portal vein. Blood goes back to the heart through the hepatic veins. The liver has a lot of blood flowing through it. If things go wrong, that's a lot of blood to lose, I remember thinking. It may have been a little flippant, but then at the time I didn't know what else to feel or think about. I could only think that I could quite easily die because of having the operation or because of not having the operation, and I didn't really like the odds either way.

Luckily, the body can cope with losing up to two-thirds of the liver. I was about to lose over 60 percent, so I was on the cusp. The reason that parts of the liver can be removed without a fatal outcome is that, uniquely, it can regenerate itself. I was assured that within three months of the operation, mine would grow back to near-normal size.

I was to have the right side of the liver removed; therefore the operation was a right hemi-hepatectomy. The gall bladder is located… guess where? Yes, the right side, which meant I was to lose that too. That part of the operation is known as a cholecystectomy.

My cancer had spread from the primary site in my gut to my liver. Without surgery, I knew the chances of surviving even five years were doubtful. A successful operation was going to improve my chance of long-term survival, but only by 30 to 40 percent. There would still be a chance of the cancer returning, even if the operation was a success. This happens in around two-thirds of all patients in my situation.

I was sent a copy of a letter that had gone to my GP. The letter explained what had happened in the meeting and what I had agreed to – to undergo a right hemi-hepatectomy. I agreed with that.

The letter said I had also agreed to a lot of other things which I didn't remember at all. So much more that I stopped reading the letter and decided I must have been in a different meeting from the rest of them.

The letter specified that there was a risk of transient liver dysfunction. However, given that my residual volume was adequate – which meant I would have just about enough liver left (40 percent) – the risk of my having acute liver insufficiency was low. It was a good job I was only copied in on the letter and that the intended reader, my GP, would undoubtedly understand it all and be ever so concerned.

Chapter 21

I was in fact to wait more than six weeks for the operation, which was delayed initially because of my episode of neutropenic sepsis over New Year. The letter I received suggested early February and a Mr S was to confirm the date after discussions with the rest of the team, no doubt at another "multidisciplinary meeting". But the surgery was delayed beyond that. Perhaps there was no CORU – or clinical operational research unit – bed available or Mr M had other more pressing and urgent cases to deal with. Either way, the operation took place on my elder sister's birthday at the end of February.

Those several weeks allowed me to rethink my life. If my discussions with Mr M were anything to go by, even with the best surgical outcome I might not have a brilliant future involving another two or three decades of active life. I didn't need to keep looking at the calendar, wondering how many days I would have to wait. I had nothing else to do except keep working on the Indian consultancy project. In the end though, nothing else was going to compete for my attention with the date. I was to be committed to the system without question and as requested. Of course I was.

Grace and I read the letter several times during that period. Due to the limited extent of our knowledge, we could perhaps start and end our discussion in one short conversation, but we did understand the risks and the potential lack of any meaningful future. We often ran through the facts together, speaking easily and freely about the technicalities of the surgery and its possible outcomes. I missed most of what other people talked about. I was thinking of dying on the table, living only for a few months at best, panicking and feeling desperate. I spent more time trying to rid myself of the dark places and that damned demon on my shoulder. The lack of sleep was grievous; it was beginning to cause me concern, as my nights were fast becoming as negative as my days.

I was very aware of trying not to get ill, because it would delay the surgery if I came down with any kind of bug, and I didn't want that. I worked in my study, mainly alone, on my client's project. I held meetings with one person from my client's company – and always the same person – at my home. I had plenty to do, plenty to keep me going and take my mind away from the dark place. The work calmed me but there were times when I would get tightly wound up and occasionally lash out with frustration, usually at Grace, for no reason except my fear had overtaken reason. Fear showed its hideous face and often spat ugly themes with contrition and hatred at me.

I tried to explain my outbursts by saying I was having a very bad time. Everything seemed to be against me. I was not going to survive. Nobody cared and nothing could be done to stop my death, but everything around me continued as before. Anger came and went and when it went it was usually replaced by morbid fear and plenty of tears – head-held-in-hands, red-eyed, deep, sobbing, woeful tears. Oh, the misery and pity that I poured on myself over those long and seemingly endless dark, cold weeks.

At times I was convinced I was going to die. Sometimes it seemed irrelevant. I would often hear myself say, *so what?* It wasn't denial, was it? I simply understood that disaster was a possible outcome and nothing would change until it was all over and I was dead and it wouldn't be a problem anymore, well not for me anyway. When that happened, others might have to deal with their own demons, their own fears and uncontrollable horrors. Nothing was going to change until it was over and I was no longer there.

But I loved my family, my wife and children and my close friends and I was loved by them, wasn't I? Being with a long-time love like Grace was like having their shape and person glued to yours with their power surging through you, passing backwards and forwards, generating and regenerating our life. I couldn't give that up. I wouldn't allow it! But I wanted someone, anyone, to tell me what to do. I wanted sympathy and at times Grace would look at me with filmy eyes, passive and afraid. I once caught her image in the mirror and saw the pain and sadness that she often hid from me during those weeks, but as I didn't open my mouth to talk I was already defeated. I needed a coach, a trainer, someone to guide me. Somebody must know how it works. After all, dying was not an unknown activity; in fact, I knew full well that it was astonishingly common.

Grace would sometimes take me out of the house. Mental preparation was always needed on those occasions. Should I or shouldn't I? I had to decide what to wear as protective amour against the cold and against illness that was outside and *lurked in other humans*. We couldn't go anywhere that was packed with people. To avoid the crowds we went to Waddesdon Manor and walked in the gardens. The house was built by Baron Rothschild in the 1870s. Today it was frosty and the light pale. The statues, covered now in white sheets and bound with string to protect them from the winter, created a ghostly, surreal atmosphere as we strolled along crunchy gravel pathways. It was good to feel the cold air on my face, breathe the cold air into my lungs. It was actually good to be alive.

Then there were days when we didn't go anywhere. I would open the shutters and see the same grey sky and not want to go out, and yet I knew that I should. So we would simply go for a walk. The day demanded it; the usual walk. Left out of the house and grounds, down through the woods and past the fields to look at the village of Chearsley, neatly settled in the next valley. Onto the flood plain, avoiding the deep, sodden areas, up and across the road and ending up behind the village by the duck pond. If we had only remembered, we would have brought some bread to feed the ducks and enjoy the brief moment before continuing on past the church, the primary school and the village hall. The village shop sometimes provided us with a teacake to burn under the grill when we got back home. It was funny how butter always made teacakes edible again after an over-grilling.

It was easy for us to stay close while we were both at home together, by each other's side on a walk or sitting together on a hill. That's when we found time to talk, I suppose. That's when we found plenty of time to discuss cancer in a more general way. Of course it existed everywhere, embodied in major and minor forms. Some people coped with it better than others, some didn't survive very long, and occasionally some sufferers lived on for many years.

The disease is often bequeathed to the dark places, to private places, kept vacuum-packed in the world of the unwell and the half dead and not discussed openly, lest it should escape and infect the light and clean places out in public. Some days we discussed the issues from dawn to dusk and then at other times we didn't talk about it at all and just held it in our minds, where it would eat away, worming deeper into the backs of our brains where the fear sat waiting to be nurtured and fed. Our discussions comforted me but often left me crying for myself and contemplation of my demise.

Grace was with me and never left my side. I wasn't allowed to eat or drink anything before we left. The demon swarmed around my head and in my ears like an angry wasp. I couldn't fight it anymore; I was beginning to give in to the inevitable outcome and the murmuring, the whisper that I was about to die. The demon told me that I would not return.

Grace drove me to the Churchill Hospital and I remember some of the journey, but I felt very distant from it all really. Reaching the outskirts of Oxford marked the divide between home and hospital and we had made this crossing many times. The Oxford college spires of learning were our test and task now. I noticed them afresh but this time was different. This time I felt them spear me in the heart. They pointed into the sky and sparkled as the sun glinted off them. These spires and college domes and church towers all refracted the light in sentinel beams, sending coloured codes soaring into the sky above. What did they mean? What did they say?

They said, *today might be your last day.*

At the Churchill Grace and I waited. We were shown to a large waiting area where we sat along with a couple of other obvious patients. The time came for me to say goodbye to her. It was a strange moment. I remember not daring to turn around to see her face as I left the room. I couldn't cope with the fact that that might be the last time I would ever see her. Not to hear her voice say goodbye was wrong. What would she do if there was a disaster? What if I died? I wasn't ready.

I was prepared in the expected and usual way, undressed and provided with a backless green gown. I had a chest x-ray and an electrocardiogram (ECG) to check my heart, I told them what medication I was taking and then had some blood tests. The whole process took a few hours. The possible negative side effects were explained again. The normal anaesthetic techniques for the procedure were a combination of general and epidural anaesthesia. The epidural was to block the nerves that supplied the area around my liver, so I was taken to a small room where I sat on a bed surrounded by students who watched my back intently as a rather large needle was inserted into me next to my spinal cord, followed by a fine tube that was to stay there, feeding my nerves with morphine for five days following the operation.

I remember rather liking morphine. At the time I wondered whether I could get it on prescription from my GP to help get rid of that little demon.

The tube into my spinal cord was very fine and I don't remember being able to feel it in my back. I was told that there was only a one-in-10,000 chance of it causing permanent nerve damage. Actually, when I thought about it, that was a 0.01-percent chance, which seemed statistically really quite high.

The anaesthetist was a young woman with cold hands and a clipped South African accent. She told me as she sank the needle deeper that, after the operation, I would be given a PCEA, which apparently stood for patient-controlled epidural analgesia. Simply put, this meant I would have a button that I could press any time I wanted more morphine and a smile on my face. The button was attached to a computerised pump that delivered the stuff though a syringe and down into the tube, to ease the pain. Thankfully there was a failsafe system to prevent me pressing away every few minutes and giving myself an overdose.

I felt very calm as I was wheeled off to the operating theatre and the last thing I remember was counting down from 10, out loud as instructed. I think I reached seven.

I awoke to find myself in an operating theatre recovery room. From there I was transferred to a high dependency unit and finally to a six-bedded, yet empty, ward. I was told that mine had been a very long operation taking several hours.

The morning after the operation, the surgeon came to see me and I just about remember him, sweeping back the curtains that still surrounded my bed and bowling up to my side. He stood there with his hands on his hips and his shirt sleeves rolled up. Around him were a group of frightened-looking, crisp-starch-white-coated, red-cheeked student doctors who followed him everywhere, note books and pens in hand.

And he said, grinning from ear to ear, "Well, Mr Brown, that was 100 percent successful. We have removed all the cancer."

This meant that, having undergone an extended right hemi-hepatectomy and a cholecystectomy, all the liver lesions had been removed, oh! along with what turned out to be not 60 but 70 percent of my liver.

It looked as though I might live to see a few more years yet.

Of course Grace came to see me as soon as was possible, as did the girls when they could get to the hospital from their places of work. We discussed the outcome, the team of surgeons and their skills and capabilities. We admired their steady, safe hands and exquisite craftsmanship. My scar was big and curved up around my body. The size of it surprised me. The sides of the wound were stapled together and stuck with glue and tape. It hurt, but only until I pressed my PCEA button.

Our conversations would often stray from the facts and the visually obvious results of the surgery to the mental ones – how I was feeling about my future now that, at least physically, the cancerous parts of my liver had been removed and the process of its own regeneration had begun, almost within hours of so much of it being taken away.

I was feeling well and Grace and I were happy being together. We had a more positive approach to our future. Yes, we expected that there would be more chemotherapy but we were thankful that I was alive. People told me I looked well for a man who had just undergone that amount of surgery, for a man who had been injected with so many terrible toxins. My weight was a little down of course, but now we could rebuild. My skin looked healthy enough and my hair was not as thin. At least it had stopped coming out when I washed it, clogging up the drain in the shower tray.

My stress level subsided. I couldn't really describe myself in words but although I didn't pay too much attention to myself physically I was conscious of how I was feeling and of my own needs, although I found it difficult to analyse. I also paid a little more attention to how I wanted to behave and respond to people and situations around me.

It was spring. The sun rose a little earlier in the mornings and woke me a little earlier each day. The spring was a joy, a blessing and a hope of a better and brighter future. It gave me an ounce more traction and bounce, like a runner wearing a better-designed pair of spiked shoes to gain an advantage on the track. I could no longer call myself unhappy and I didn't want to spin the story of death and loss anymore. Although my thoughts were still a little ragged, like shifting and reforming clouds, to consider surviving was as clear and as refreshing as the blue sky that provided the backdrop to those clouds. Up there where the air was thinner it made me heady with happiness. Survival meant survival for all of us and our future programme was to fight, to fly up into the blue skies that had suddenly appeared above us, and help colour and paint a new canvas.

There was nothing now to be angry about and everything to play for. A new template of happier times was being developed and, although yet to be formalised, was indeed being formed. The good was now rising to the surface to become a natant layer of happiness and I was becoming part of the floating upper layer, bobbing on the surface and becoming impressively more active and optimistic.

As the pressure was eased, so the realisation grew that I could live again. Was there now a chance to be optimistic? Could we now seek out those slivers of silver hope? We couldn't have adopted optimism before. It had to be real, tangible and ours, and now it seemed it could be. It wasn't necessarily going to be easy nor without doubt or possible pitfalls, but it was there, not to be got rid of or thrown away. It was appropriate and it wasn't embarrassing. We really did have optimism about the outcome after all this time.

We became blessings counters.

Grace was gifted with balance as well as ballast. My sturdy, steady rock could now help me stabilise my life and help me understand the physical sense of just being in this world with the sun on my face, to smell the earth and see the light and once more connect with the people I loved and love still. My landscape was opening again before me; the three dimensions of its shape were reforming in front of me and becoming fixed underneath the brightening skies.

I started to see new things being built and mountains readjusting their size, growing larger and more beautiful and majestic. Outcrops turned from greys to greens, promontories began to glow with colour. From my new vantage point I was viewing the world from a much better angle. I understood it without effort or hazy vision. It was becoming the new view that I had of the very stuff of life itself.

As my new liver started to grow, so did my desire to go home. I wanted to get back to my normality, see my friends and family. The surgical clips holding my wound together were beginning to hurt now despite the morphine. One three-inch section seemed not to be healing well at all. The food in the Churchill could have been better, but I had tasted worse. The staff were always quietly efficient and the doctors and consultants clinical.

Two days after entering the ward I was joined by another, similarly-aged patient. Apart from his age, a greying moustache and silver-framed reading glasses, he reminded me instantly of Del Trotter in the comedy *Only Fools and Horses*. He had a mobile phone permanently glued to his right ear, several gold rings on as many fingers and a wonderfully rich South-London accent. He spent most of his time pacing backwards and forward around the ward talking earnestly on his phone, his dressing gown open to the waist to show off the large medallion that hung around his neck, setting off the horizontally-stapled scar that he also bore as the result of a similar liver operation to mine. He was a chipper chappie, especially when his daughter came to see him, which she did daily, usually in the early afternoon and always accompanied with loud raucous laughter, a box of well appreciated but probably forbidden chocolates and, on one occasion, a small but obvious hip flask of Johnnie Walker Black Label whisky.

We chatted to each other as patients do, especially when there are only two of them alone in a ward. The nurses were not around and, unusually, the man's TV was not showing the latest horseracing results. He delighted in telling me that his big silver Mercedes was bigger than my car, his 60-inch flat-screen TV was bigger than mine and his two Irish greyhounds were both bigger than my dog Charlie. He did admit though that his daughter wasn't a true blonde, he fancied my wife and his son was "well, he's in the theatre business, doesn't like girls and lives in Brighton."

Grace and I met both his daughter and, indeed, on a couple of occasions, his son. The latter arrived one evening, was greeted with a gruff *how're you?* from his father and was then left to sit by his father's side. The son was dressed very elegantly, all in black – black leather gloves, thick woollen Crombie coat and black silk scarf. He thumbed through a slim paperback with his gloves on while his father watched the TV. I caught the son's eye once or twice and he would smile before returning to his book. The second time he came to visit, he came over to me and asked if I would like a cup of tea as he was making one for his father. I accepted and he smiled. I suddenly felt very sorry for him. He obviously loved his father and yet they were so much at the opposite ends of life's spectrum that it must have been painful, no doubt for both of them.

The son offered to pick his father up the following day as he was being discharged. Despite having no alternative at the time, the old man vehemently declined this offer. Once his son had left the ward after his visit, my fellow patient shouted across to me, "Sorry abaht me son, Dave, but I can't really 'ave '*im* take me 'ome, now can I?"

In all, I spent seven days after my operation on the ward before being discharged on 5 March.

Chapter 22

Two days after I was discharged the district nurse came to our house to remove the surgical clips. The wound had mostly healed well, apart from what was now a deep and infected two-inch gash on my right side, below the last rib. I had regular visits from the nurse after that and on each occasion she cleaned and redressed the wound but it still wouldn't heal.

Three weeks later I was due to have a chest x-ray and a check-up of my wound. My post-operative recovery was being marred by the infected wound complication so I was to be seen by a doctor. Grace was with me in a small anteroom. Two young doctors arrived and immediately began to interrogate me, notes in hand, before telling me to strip to the waist, lie on the trolley bed and keep still. They drew the curtain around us and, without another word, picked up a pair of six-inch forceps, opened up the wound and with several wads of cotton wool, cleaned out the pus, re packed it and slapped a sticking plaster over it.

I think Grace nearly fainted when she heard my screams in response to what I can honestly say was a rather painful experience. Despite their arrogant and unacceptably poor bedside manner, lack of personal sensitivity and refusal to use an anaesthetic, their quick, in-and-out, brutal assault worked wonderfully and within another week or so the wound started to heal at last. With that, I was signed off from the Churchill Hospital with the hope that the wound would cause no further problems. They gave me a letter to my GP explaining the situation and requesting that I have a CT scan in six months, followed by an annual scan for the next five years.

My liver was re-growing briskly. The risk of lesions recurring on my new liver was explained to me again by the surgeon Mr R, and I was therefore referred back to my oncologist Dr J to discuss the options of further chemotherapy as well as for her to follow my progress over the following five years.

I became mobile again as quickly as I possibly could and ate as much as the caterers could bring me. The epidural pain-controlling morphine arrangement PCEA had sadly been stepped down. Pain control was now to consist of an oral analgesic on the fifth day, three days before I was sent home.

At the same time that the epidural was removed I developed what was at first thought to be a chest infection but turned out to be iatrogenic pneumothorax, which in plain language meant I had a small amount of air in the cavity around my right lung, caused by the insertion of a central line during the operation. Although this was initially a concern to the medics, it resolved itself sufficiently for me to be signed off eight days after the operation, provided I had a chest x-ray three weeks later to make sure the air bubble had gone.

The surgical team were happy with the results of the operation and indeed my recovery on the ward. I had the usual painkillers prescribed but I needed to inject myself daily with dalteparin for a further 20 days to protect myself against blood clots. I came to appreciate what diabetics go through when they have to inject themselves with insulin regularly.

There were times when I was in pain. The peripheral neuropathy was always there but not getting worse; it was the liver surgery wound and sometime my stoma that hurt.

I lost track of the drugs I was taking. I needed to eat food with some and drink water with others. The regime would start at 8.00 am as I was pitched from sleep into a world of drug taking. Grace watched me sometimes to make sure I took all my medicines and watched the little bit of milk drip off my lip and down my front. Would all mornings be like this now? I would grip my mug of tea and take the next pill.

Finally, I would dump myself on a sofa, armatured and buttressed with cushions. I would sit like a grand Buddha, commanding the world around me. Slowly, the sofa became less necessary and as the pain eased and the scars healed, so did my mind. Grace would lean against my shoulder and we would relax together and enjoy each other's company as we used to do before. I had been gifted, she told me, even though there had been some changes to my life. I had my life back. I had the gift given back. We were not to think of pity or sorrow anymore; sadness maybe and a sort of intractable physical weight at the unsavoury hand we had been dealt, but not pity. This was us now. How could I feel pity for myself? Seen from many other people's perspective we were great and I should feel lucky to be alive. And I was! So this was how it was going to be.

March and April were months of recuperation after the liver operation and it was time that allowed me to start work again, although I wasn't going to be travelling back to India or indeed anywhere overseas until my wound had properly healed. Raj, my link to the work that was progressing all across India now, came to visit me on a regular basis and we would work in my study, drinking copious amounts of tea, dealing with all the issues and developing future programmes for the team in Bangalore. Raj would bring little presents of Indian sweets that his wife had kindly made, and sometimes flowers for Grace. He was my contact with the outside business world. The work he represented was welcome and necessary for my recovery on so many levels.

Al, one of my dearest friends, would also drop by and on occasion we would go for a beer, walking up to the village pub where he would, as always, listen to my world of woes and work issues and, as always, provide me with alternative thoughts on dealing with the issues with which I presented him. He was always there for me, always without condemnation, always with a practical and objective potential solution and always a joy to be with. Indeed, he still is.

I was due to see Dr J in mid-April as a new round of chemotherapy was going to start as soon as I was healthy enough. This was planned for May. Dr J wasn't there on the 15th, the day of my appointment, as she was on vacation with her family, so instead for the first time we met Dr J's specialist registrar, Dr O. It was a strange encounter. There was no balance to the meeting. We couldn't look forwards to my further recovery, nor backwards to the early days of my illness, as he had little knowledge about what had happened in my story to bring me to this point. He had to read my medical notes each time he spoke, which seemed to take an age. Even having briefed himself, he didn't really seem to understand my medical history. Also, he wasn't as engaging as Dr J, so there was very little personal interaction, nor did it seem there was going to be. Dr O was, for me, just Dr J's stand in. He might as well have given me a flysheet or a memo on a piece of A4 paper or sent an email to my laptop.

It made me realise just how central Dr J had become in our world. She was our fulcrum and had been all the way through those first precarious days. She provided an immense amount of support, care and knowledge. I missed her that day. I missed her lovely eyes and warm rhetoric. I missed her caring tone and carefully expressed knowledge that had always made me feel safe, even when I knew I wasn't.

I was assigned nurses who came to the house to help with dressings and check my wound before and after the brutal doctors' intervention. I was managing my stoma, although sometimes I was still caught short after eating something that changed the timings, altered the routine or just caused an upset. The loperamide usually helped, but even that faithful drug let me down on occasions.

I was not always impressed by the nurses' training or remit. They never stayed long, 15 minutes or so; they were always late in arriving. There was never any time to get to know them, but then what would have been the point? They had so many other patients to see and some needed more attention than others. I gained the impression that my needs were the least important to them. Nor did I want to waste their time. On the positive side, the nurses' visits made a jolly mid-morning interlude and it was reassuring always to have a second opinion about my physical progress.

In the end it became clear that I didn't need professional home care any longer and we brought an end to the nurses' visits, once they were happy that I could take proper care of myself. I was no longer feeling under attack or feeling vulnerable.

Cancer no longer did that to me.

Chapter 23

When we visited Dr O in Dr J's oncology clinic in April, I had to tell him that the hemi-hepatectomy and cholecystectomy procedures had been successful and that the surgeons reckoned they had resected all outbreaks of the disease. I could have made it up but nevertheless he related my account in a letter to my GP. He and Dr J had discussed my situation and the rationale for further chemotherapy. There was no clear reason for more drug treatment. However, given the fact that the disease had recurred in my liver after the bowel cancer – despite adjuvant chemotherapy – they recommended further chemo treatment to reduce the possibility of another recurrence. The number of cycles hadn't been decided, but a new PICC line was to be inserted.

I was due to go to India for two weeks to continue the work Raj and I had been developing, so I persuaded the medics to delay the start of my course until the latter part of May.

On 20 May I was back at the Stoke Mandeville cancer clinic. A new PICC line was inserted and, after another few hours sitting in a brightly-coloured plastic armchair being infused with the latest cocktail of drugs, a new pump was strapped around my waist.

This treatment cycle was called cycle five. It was to be a continuation of the programme I had left off several months before. A further six or seven cycles were planned after cycle five.

The nursing staff I encountered when I returned to the clinic were more or less as I remembered; the same smiling faces and busy schedules. Philip was there with his wide grin, vast show of white teeth and glowing smile.

"Welcome back, Mr Brown."

What did he think this was, a spa hotel? Was I back for another long relaxing holiday, lounging around in comfy electric armchairs, drinking warm orange juice and munching cheese and pickle sandwiches, followed by fruit yoghurts (with very little fruit), while nurses stuck needles in my arms and drip-fed highly expensive, transparent liquids directly into my heart and I met, conversed with and eyeballed the other holiday-makers?

The best nurses there were efficient and were always capable of assessing situations quickly and easily. They received my instant praise to their patron saint. One or two could quickly identify those patients who needed immediate attention, those who were in pain and those who just needed a hand held or a friendly smile and a few words. Some nurses would work together on a patient who might have concerns or fears. I watched them with admiration in the unspoken, silent, efficient way they went about their tasks. One wonderful nurse had the habit of talking almost continuously, dispensing the pure tonic of talk. To me it was like a stream of nitrogen bubbles in a pint of Guinness, but to many of her patients it was the heavenly bubbles of life. Even as I watched her I could see the patients around her raising their tired heads to smile. Everywhere she went she created a resurgence of hope and light.

The pump I was given was a new design, made in China. I wondered what the reason was for the change. Cost reduction was my immediate thought. The reason for mentioning this is because of what happened the night I got home from my second session during the first week of June.

My peripheral neuropathy had started to get worse again, this time in my feet. I now spent many minutes every night "cycling" under the duvet. Grace found it impossible to sleep with me when I thrashed around like this and exiled me to the top floor bedroom, which was not as bad as it sounds because the top floor is really another guest suite, with a big bed and a shower.

As before, I found sleeping with the pump around my waist an inconvenient annoyance. If I slipped it under the pillow it was more comfortable and helped ensure that I didn't pull the PICC line out of my arm. With the warmer nights and early morning light, I found sleeping was generally requiring a bigger effort. There was a bird outside the window that woke me early every morning as the sun rose, which in June meant very early. I had no idea what kind of bird it was, but I loved its varied and crystal-clear repertoire. It was my dear friend Al who eventually enlightened me as to the species, drawing from his "twitcher" knowledge; otherwise I wouldn't have had a clue. It was a robin, he said. The robin's melodies drowned out all other bird song, in fact all other sound really. He must have perched in the same place each morning until his mate finally arrived and responded, at which point he would disappear and the chorus would cease.

His song made me smile every time and, despite being exiled to the top floor, I was happy and could see my future start to rise again like a phoenix out of the cancerous ashes in which I had waded about for so long.

The pump was designed to deliver a finite quantity of drugs into my bloodstream over each period of 24 hours. I would put it on as I left the clinic and spend the next two days at home. When the pump was empty, a couple of days later, I would drop by the clinic again and have it removed, my PICC tube flushed out and the dressing changed. Part of this was to check my arm for any sign of inflammation that would suggest infection. It was the same process as when I first had a PICC line.

When I used this new pump, with its new design, I noticed that the drugs ran out several hours before they were supposed to. The down-side of this is obvious in that it meant I had been given the chemotherapy drugs at a faster rate than intended, potentially creating a dangerous overdose. Frantic phone calls and an immediate visit to the clinic ensued. I was examined thoroughly and found to be OK, not perilously poisoned.

I was told I must have got the timings wrong when the drip feed had finished. I was not pleased with this response and started to work out the flow rates to determine the exact dosage. I researched the design and technology of the pump and discovered what I could about the manufacturer. I was horrified to learn that the accuracy of this pump, and indeed of most other pump designs, was plus or minus up to 10 percent. Worse still, nobody I could find at the clinic or at the manufacturing company cared – not the nurses, doctors or oncologists. The hospital's pharmacy department was given the task of investigating the problem. They didn't.

The rest of June and July was taken up with the ongoing chemotherapy cycles, two in June and three more in July. I saw Dr J in both June and mid-July to discuss my progress. Consultancy work for my Indian client was coming to an end. There were new procedures to be developed, but I was doing that from the UK. The whole project was finally going to be completed before the autumn.

When Grace and I saw Dr J in June for a review, it was just before my third cycle of the new chemotherapy regime. I had made an excellent recovery from the liver resection, she told me with her usual sparkle. My performance status was still zero – which was good. The two drugs, irinotecan and fluorouracil, seemed to be having little toxic effect which was also considered good.

The remaining problem was still the peripheral neuropathy in my feet and especially my toes, caused when I was taking the oxaliplatin. I had been put on amitriptyline and the dose was increased twice. Although I seemed to respond positively to the larger dose, My feet and toes were still painful and were not getting any better with time. I had also developed a rash on my chest and back and whilst Dr J wasn't too concerned about this, she did give me a wrinkled-brow look which I hadn't seen before. I was offered duloxetine as an alternative drug, which I started taking in July.

My local GP surgery continued to surprise me with its constant written rhetoric and yet total lack of follow-through. No GP had come to see me since my medical troubles began. I was

147

supposedly under a Dr W and yet, at the end of July, a letter arrived telling me how a new service was to be set up for "people who are more at risk of an unplanned hospital admission in an emergency situation". I had had three unplanned hospital admissions already and not once had my local GP clinic even been aware. The letter continued with its inane drivel about how I would be "likely to benefit from more tailored, active support from your GP surgery". I nearly exploded with fury. It was amazing how three usually positive and proactive words could be used in a sentence that so far in all my dealings with my local surgery had been the opposite. Tailored? Yes to ignoring me. Active support? Apart from the 70-year-old locum doctor – without whose suspicions and fast actions in sending me to A&E right at the beginning, I might well have died – there had been little support and certainly nothing that I could vaguely describe as being *active*. The letter went on to inform me that "my named GP will work with you to develop a personal care plan and review". My named doctor, (a different) Dr W, has never contacted me. I still have no personal care plan and all the copies of letters to and from the clinic are to the original Dr W.

I hoped that the practice manager at my local health centre was just having a bad day when she wrote that letter, but I have my doubts.

I reached a landmark – my last chemotherapy treatment, followed by a farewell to the inaccurate pump. The removal of the PICC line was to be the last active violation of my body by the chemotherapy nursing staff and, although the catheter was quickly and expertly removed, the occasion still brought a tear to my eye.

This was not because it was the final act after all the surgery, radiotherapy and chemotherapy to treat my cancer, but because it damn well hurt.

Suddenly I felt vulnerable and uncared for. I had been "in the system" for two years and now I was being jettisoned back out into real life without my overseers. Yes, I would have my faithful Dr J and of course Grace and the girls, but the system was moving me out and replacing me with other needy patients. Of course they now needed the facilities that ultimately had saved me, but I was feeling disturbed. I wanted to just run away to work it all out somewhere, leave the car, catch a bus to some destination and hide out for a while. That was the odd thing – that I wanted to stay in the hospital and yet escape from it forever. I was mobile and had autonomy so I could have run. I wondered how many other post-treatment patients had felt as I did then. The institution was the whole apparatus of medical practice that made me better, held me together, and looked after me.

I sat there in my plastic armchair in number three bay in the Stoke Mandeville cancer clinic with my cup of weak coffee and thought about the moment. It was here that I seemed to have spent a lot of my recent life. I looked around. There were no spaces. Hospitals hate voids. Spaces need to be filled, if not with equipment then with people. Hospitals seem to strive against entropy. The three bays in the clinic had excess chairs for visitors, stacked up in corners in a way that seemed to make it impossible for the average visitor to grapple one free. There were side tables everywhere that made it difficult for staff to negotiate their way through the clinic quickly, as sometimes they needed to. Patients' wheelchairs and zimmer frames just made things worse by creating less space and more obstacles to fall over.

Most of the nurses had seemed to zip easily around these hurdles in the past, hadn't they? Or maybe I just hadn't noticed. It was probably why they were all so trim; probably good at Zumba too. I suddenly noticed the harsh lighting again, fluorescent tubes in plastic holders that helped illuminate the old, sad pictures that lined the walls. I had never really looked at them before. Why would I have done? I thought. They were prints of flowers, giant chrysanthemums, poppies and roses that without doubt had been there for several years.

As it was a hot day, the rear exit door was propped open with one of the many spare visitors' chairs. They had *some* use then. The breeze was comforting for most people but one elderly lady was getting a nasty draught on her left side. She complained about the open door but was out-voted.

Sitting there at that moment suddenly helped me realise that in some small way it was pay-back time. I wanted to make the nurses' lives easier. I wanted to ensure that there were always enough plastic armchairs, so patients wouldn't be turned away or have to wait. I wanted the experience at this chemotherapy clinic to be as good as it was at the hospital in Oxford, where I had been filled with so much hope and received such feelings of wellbeing. Just the sense that you are really being cared for is an amazing healer. That I mattered and people wanted to help me get better had been vitally important to me, looking back. I stared again at the pictures on the walls and chairs around the room and the room itself. A nurse asked me if I was alright as the single tear on my cheek had been joined by more. "It was the PICC line," I lied. She squeezed my hand and smiled before rushing off to drape a woollen blanket on the lap of the old lady with a draught on her side.

I decided that I needed to donate something. A new electric clinical chair would cost just under £2,000 and an original painting produced for one of the bays, by an internationally known RSA artist, would be well in excess of £5,000.

But one by yours truly? Just a decent-sized canvas and a few dabs of oil paint?

Chapter 24

That summer was a busy one for the family. Emily was completing her doctorate and her fiancé Ben was doing the same as well as running his successfully growing business. The twins had developing careers. Harriet was now working for the charity Cancer Research UK, having been awarded her second degree, this time in marketing. Alice was blazing a trail in the Middle East with an American engineering company.

The year before, over lunch and three pints of good ale at my local village pub one lunch time, Ben had finally asked me for Emily's hand in marriage, and now the wedding was planned for the coming autumn. Emily and Ben chose 2 October for their wedding, the same day as Grace's and mine and indeed my parents' before us. Needless to say, my mum and dad would have been pleased; I was pleased too, mainly because I was alive and could actually be there. Hurray!

Although I knew that I wanted to paint something for the clinic, I couldn't get any appropriate subjects into place in my head. I knew it would happen but I wasn't sure when.

I regularly received information from Cancer Research UK and learned this way that they were organising an event that summer, a nationwide barbecue one weekend in July. Joining this great event locally would be an opportunity to gather friends, family and neighbours together. I hatched the idea of hosting our own event and persuading our guests to donate generously towards the worthy cause of cancer research.

I wanted the occasion to be a fun day out for everyone, with games as well as traditional barbecue food, and I knew my dearest friend and superb games master, Al, would again help. He did. My intention was to make the day easy to manage, requiring only light work, banal and beautifully boring. Although Al had other ideas.

Before the weekend of the barbecue, on a gloriously sunny day, Grace and I drove over from our seaside retreat to spend a day at Chartwell House in Kent. Chartwell was of course the principal home of Sir Winston Churchill and his wife Clementine and still sits beautifully in rolling hills a couple of miles south of Westerham. Run efficiently by the National Trust now, it was a perfect outing for us as we both love the properties that NT cares for around the country, and especially wanted to see the gardens in full bloom.

Wandering through the gardens was wonderful. We passed through elegant brick arches covered in early blossoming roses, beneath the high walls and along the cold frames, through greenhouses, orchards and fruit gardens. We sat on a bench at the back of the house with a late afternoon cuppa. It was four o'clock and the light was changing as the sun sank towards late afternoon.

The gardeners were still at their work. As I watched them, I realised that their toil represented a truly artistic, and historic, combination of tasks. These gardeners still maintained the Chartwell grounds as they and others before them had done for many decades. A multitude of rough-skinned hands had tended those same beds for a century. Horticultural capability at its best was there for all to see and admire. The pathway edges were immaculately finished, allowing the grass to slope away like green carpet, clipped to perfection. York-stone lanes stopped neatly by steps at the gates up to the house. The earth in the beds was madly fertile, fed with high-grade mulch that increased its potency. I spied many different varieties of fruits, from Williams pear and quince to Honeycrisp apple and copious types of plum. I could have spent hours in that spectacular place. There was a climbing clump of flowering *Clematis montana* and Indigoletta roses, alongside bushes of Clotted Cream jasmine.

The walled staircase was dripping with Virginia creeper, its leaves not yet their spectacular deep, orange-fired red. Climbing hydrangeas stood like erect soldiers against the walls. The afternoon light was stunning and the various flowering shrubs glowed in that light as the gardeners began to pack up for the day. One by one, they put down their spades and forks, placed their brooms into the wheelbarrows, stretched their aching backs and pulled off their soiled gloves.

We could hear them chatting and laughing. They smiled at each other as they cleared away their tools. Happy and contented, they patted each other's shoulders and briefly draped their arms around another in comradeship. Another day of toil yes, but also another day of nurturing new plants to grow and thrive, another day of sowing fresh seed to sprout and grow, and another day of pruning away dead wood, dead leaves, dead cells to allow new healthy growth to develop.

Here, in front of me, were a team of wonderfully capable and dedicated, skilled people who were bringing new life back to that garden every day, every month and every year, for as long as the garden existed. They were the chemotherapy and radiotherapy nurses and the doctors and my consultant oncologist who did the same for me and for so many other patients every day at the clinic. They were the team who had nurtured me back to life, who had helped clear away the dead, cancerous cells to give me a new start, a new shot at life. These gardeners would therefore be perfect as the study for a picture that I would paint for the Stoke Mandeville cancer clinic.

The world experienced is the world described. I started to take a series of photographs of each of the gardeners as they finished their digging and sweeping, clearing away the tools. It was a happy moment and I felt pleased that I had been there to witness the moment and take from it the inspiration that I hoped I could use to create my own form of thanks to the hospital and inspiration for others.

I received the Cancer Research UK barbecue organisers' pack. It contained information posters and some barbecue paraphernalia. I was feeling extremely good about this and looked forward to preparing for the day. Al and I agreed the games to be played and the size of the teams, based on those who were due to come. We erected a marquee on the back lawn to accommodate both some of the games as well as a makeshift bar.

We set up the barbecue itself and surrounded it with as many chairs, tables and sun umbrellas as we possessed. We marked out places for the various outdoor games to be played. It was like a boys' camping weekend, except we had girls coming as well.

The day turned out to be not only one of the warmest but also one of the sunniest that year. The games took effort to prepare, organise and manage, to ensure that everyone had a good time, but they were a great success.

The barbecue area was of course where most people spent most of their time, except when they weren't at the bar or being dragooned into active participation in whichever game was next on the agenda. Being at home in my own garden and cooking and eating together with all the friends and family who had supported me along my terrible journey thus far was probably one of the most important times in my recent life. It decorated my day, a day that was somehow a very different day to those gone by.

It was a greedy day, of carcinogenically-prepared sausages and burgers, copious amounts of chilled Pinot Noir and summer ales, a day of excess. Excess food and drink of course, but also a day of excess love and friendship, excess fun in the games we all played and exchanges of thanks. The plates were large ones that day and the glasses full ones. The sun was warm, the temperature perfect and once the last sausage had been burnt and the last game played, I found myself standing in the corner of the garden underneath the heavy, dark canopy of our oversized horse chestnut tree and smiling with thanks for all those who had come to share the occasion and who had helped me in my time of trouble, and indeed for all of those that weren't there too. Although I felt the tears well up in my eyes, it wasn't because of the demon that day. He had been banished, for the time being anyway.

When we counted it all, we found we had raised a substantial amount of money for CRUK that I am sure we were all very proud of. We had enjoyed a good time, we had rejoiced in my renewed health, we had toasted the nurses, doctors and Dr J but we had also taken a new stand. A stand for life. And so, as a final act that day, we collectively painted four pictures.

I had bought four blank canvases and drawn on them an outline depiction of our CRUK barbecue day. I now invited everyone present at the event to fill in any part of any drawing in any colour on the canvas of their choice. The outlines I'd done to start them off were bold depictions and had relationships with each other: the first three showed a burger, a face and a nurse, while the fourth was a game and a message of hope and thanks. They started as pencil pictograms and now, after all the guests had contributed to the artistic process, they were brightly coloured with acrylic paint. This was unlike anything any of my friends and family had done before. I watched them concentrate as they painted, desperately trying to stay within the drawn lines, using colours to emphasise a personal point.

It was my gift to both them and to me. As the party drew to a close, we all stood around the canvases, pushing them together to form one large painting of an exceptional day. I spoke a few words as one does, but I was overwhelmed by the silence as everyone gazed on *their own accomplishment*, the work they had done in supporting and helping me was all there on those four collated canvases, that collective painting of hope for the future.

I am proud of the photograph I still have of us all, with our last glasses raised to our own big composite picture on that wonderfully sunny day in July.

Chapter 25

Although Emily's and Ben's wedding wasn't for another couple of months, there seemed to be a lot going on. I had decided to back off from my consultancy work to allow Grace and me more time together and maybe a little more vacation time too. Yet we were busy with a multitude of jobs that over the past two years of our lives had just been put on hold. I was feeling well but I knew that I was still on the hook and it began to tell on me when I received a date for my next CT scan. The letter called me for an appointment in November.

Even that far away I knew that I was never going to be totally free of the threats and fears that were still hanging over me. Yes, I was alive and very grateful to be so. Yes, I had been given a second chance to enjoy that life with my family and friends, but I would always have to be monitored. My stoma was not only a daily but a minute-by-minute reminder of what had happened and what I had been through. I wasn't complaining. I wasn't ungrateful, not at all. But I was – and still am – very aware of how close to death I came, how easy it is to lose the precious life we have all been blessed with, how amazingly skilled and caring this country's doctors and nurses are and, above all, how much I love my family – my wife and adorable children and their new families – and how much I thank them and all my true friends who supported me all the way.

All this didn't take away the dread that my next medical appointment stirred up in me. Of course it wasn't the scan that was the issue, it was the result that I feared, the result that could reveal that the cancer had returned – perhaps to the same places, perhaps to somewhere else – and in so doing would halt me in my tracks and send me back to the dark place from where I would have to start all over again.

I decided to start the Chartwell canvas with the intent of completing it before Emily's wedding. It took several attempts to get all my figures in the right positions so that the composition worked. The canvas wasn't very big, just 100 by 80cm, the right sort of size to fit in the corridor of the clinic if that was where I could persuade them to hang it. The colours needed to be bold and strong, I decided. Sitting in my studio in front of a blank canvas on the easel is sometimes daunting, but with the knowledge of exactly what I wanted to get into the space, it seemed easy that morning. It was a radiant summer's morning and light filled the room. My new future, my chance at a new beginning, was going to saturate the canvas, and in the painting I hoped I would provide some anticipation of a new chance and a new beginning for others too.

The figures started to take shape with clear outlines. There would be a beginning and an end in the work. I busied myself for hours, head buried close to determine the detail. My hand was firm and the shapes developed with ease and certainty. The background shades took time. How deep to make the greens and how pale the blues? I found the shades becoming more difficult and I struggled to create the right tones, the one that I had fixed in my mind. I chose colours that were deep and saturating, to soak up the senses that would strike viewers of the finished picture with purpose and definition.

Those days I spent working on the picture I was an artist. Painting was an art and a skill that felt easily within my reach to develop as I wanted. The ideas flowed freely and galloped ahead of my ability to paint, like a springer spaniel straining at the leash. My painting started to take on its own personality. Every time I went back to look at it or add another stroke, it developed more character. There were no pale ice-cream colours here, but strong, bold, energising colours like acid lime and deep strawberry, turquoise and sienna. The early evening sunlight in summer across the garden scene was taking shape, morphing as it grew. The painting was neither clever nor witty, but it told the simple story of new growth tended by skilled and careful gardeners who nurtured living plants.

Suddenly one morning, as I stood in the doorway of the studio with the smell of oils and white spirit still rising from the canvas, I knew it was finished. I smiled, relieved. Everything I wanted to say was now there on canvas.

It was done.

When the day came to present the painting to the Stoke Mandeville cancer clinic I wanted Dr J to see it first. I wanted to give it to her. I wanted her to understand that it was as much for her as for the nursing staff. I felt pleased when it was hung at the end of the corridor for patients and staff alike to see as they walked to and from the chemotherapy bays where the treatment took place.

Donating money to the clinic to say thank you to the staff proved slightly more difficult to arrange than giving a painting, but in the end I was pleased that although some went for a new clinic chair and some for training, we made sure that half would be used for a slap-up Christmas party dinner out for the staff.

The day of the wedding came sooner than I had anticipated. Emily and Ben worked relentlessly to ensure that everything was precisely managed, so making it as painless as possible for Grace and me. All the friends and family that I loved were going to be there.

Obviously, this definition would have included all the medics who had helped me survive. But this was a family occasion and they wouldn't have wanted to come. Still, as I waited for my daughter, I remember thinking that without those other people I wouldn't have been standing there at all.

Emily took my arm and together we walked up between the line of maple trees, into the barn and up the aisle. Together we swished between my congregated friends and family. The atmosphere was electric. I was alive and so happy.

My brother jumped out into the space between the rows of guests, camcorder in hand, grinning as he filmed. I looked at Emily briefly. She was radiant, happy and smiling. I too was happy and smiled back at my brother's lens as he crouched, trying to look professional, to get the right shot. As we got closer to him, he stepped back into his seat and as we passed him I heard him say, "I haven't seen David looking so happy for many, many months."

My coat-hanger smile widened but, as I looked to my left to see where he was, I just caught a glimpse of a dark shadow sitting on my shoulder, hardly visible but nevertheless there. And the fog descended and the treacle returned and I could just see the demon eyes and the twisted smile.

Just in time I turned to look at Emily one more time as we reached the end of the rows of seats. Emily's future husband turned to take her hand. I let go of her arm and bowed my head.

Help Pages

Here I have tried to distil my whole experience of cancer into a few key points that might help others who find themselves going through the same processes as my family, friends and I did.

1) When you go to an appointment, you may not immediately understand, or later remember, everything that's said, particularly if it's bad news. Take someone else along, armed with pen and paper, and ask them to take notes.
2) Be prepared for medical professionals who are not always sympathetic. Although they may be trained in adopting a "bedside manner", they still prefer to deal with facts and figures than with emotional issues.
3) Medics deal with probability not certainty. They can't tell you what will happen after this or that intervention, or after none; only the likelihood of what may happen, based on similar cases in the past.
4) Prepare for your meetings with consultants, doctors and even nurses. Write down your questions and concerns beforehand. If you give them a copy before the meeting they will be able to

prepare answers, making the meeting shorter and more productive.

5) Lean on loved ones who offer support. Navigating your way around cancer can be very traumatic, and best not done alone.

6) Find the consultant who is best for you, someone you can trust and feel comfortable with. Not every patient has much choice, but don't be "done to"; you deserve to have your say.

The Paintings

I am an enthusiastic amateur when it comes to painting, but having enjoyed the luxury of travel to many wonderful places around the world, I have been able to capture images from some beautiful locations in England and overseas.

With only a GCE qualification in art from school and no formal training, I started to paint in the late 1990s and now work in both oil and watercolour, exhibiting two or three times a year locally in Buckinghamshire. I sell my work through exhibitions, commissions and online.

Some of my pictures can be viewed and purchased from my website: www.sorrellart123.com

Dune Fence

Oil on canvas by David I Brown

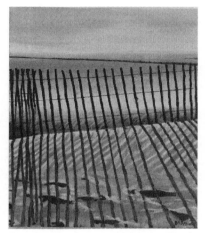

The inspiration for this picture came while I was sitting one day on an isolated beach in Queensland, Australia. Although many artists have painted similar types of scenes and many people have suffered cancer, for me this is the scene that supports my story. *Dune Fence* depicts two key images. The first is the fence, which is the barrier that was my cancer, while the second is the blue open sky and sea and a clear horizon. This is my future and the ever-present hope of beating cancer. The fence can always be surmounted.

My wife won't let me sell this painting; she keeps it prominently displayed at home to remind her of our successful fight together against cancer.

Spring Gardeners – Caring for a New Beginning

Oil on canvas by David I Brown

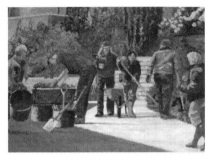

I painted this picture after watching gardeners at Chartwell House as they were finishing work for the evening in late spring near the end of my treatment. I thought the combination of activities that summarised the day's work and the new planting they had just completed provided a perfect study.

I presented the picture to my oncologist Dr J in March 2015 for the staff and patients, present and future, of the Stoke Mandeville cancer clinic. My personal experience was that recovery can be aided by hope and I would be delighted if my painting could, in some small way, help instil such a feeling in other patients. The gift was also to thank the chemotherapy staff for their wonderful support during my treatment when my life was in their skilled hands.

The Author

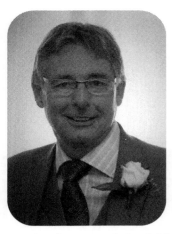

David I Brown was born in 1953 and was educated in London. He spent his early career working for large global manufacturing businesses, which took him to many places around the world. Later, he started his own consultancy in risk management, continuing to travel widely. His business and travel, particularly in India where he made many eye-opening journeys, helped him keep focused when in middle age he discovered he had a life-threatening cancer.

He has been married to Grace since 1981, has three grown-up daughters and is now a semi-retired grandfather. He and his wife live in Buckinghamshire, England, spending time at their seaside retreat on the West Sussex coast and travelling further afield whenever possible.

23126176R00101

Printed in Great Britain
by Amazon